CANCER OF THE OESOPHAGUS

CLINICAL CANCER MONOGRAPHS
Volume 1

Cancer of the Oesophagus

Hugoe R. Matthews, FRCS
Regional Department of Thoracic Surgery
East Birmingham Hospital
Birmingham B9 5ST

and

John A.H. Waterhouse, MA, PhD, HonFFOM
Jean Powell, BSc, FIS
Janet E. Robertson, BA
Christopher C. McConkey, BSc
Regional Cancer Registry
Queen Elizabeth Medical Centre
Birmingham B15 2TH

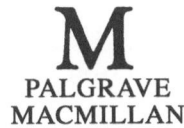

PALGRAVE
MACMILLAN

First published 1987

Published by
THE MACMILLAN PRESS LTD
Houndmills, Basingstoke, Hampshire RG21 2XS
and London
Companies and representatives
throughout the world

ISBN 978-1-349-09076-1   ISBN 978-1-349-09074-7
DOI 10.1007/978-1-349-09074-7

Library of Congress Cataloging-in-Publication Data
Matthews, Hugoe R.
Cancer of the oesophagus.
(Clinical cancer monographs; v. 1)
Bibliography: p.
1. Esophagus—Cancer—England—West Midlands—
Statistics. 2. Esophagus—Cancer—Treatment—England—
West Midlands—Statistics. I. Title. II. Series.
[DNLM: 1. Esophageal Neoplasms—occurrence—Great
Britain. WI 250 M439c]
RC280.E8M38   1987   362.1'9699'432   87–1910
ISBN 978-0-935859-09-6

Contents

Foreword

Although it is now some fifty years since the first successful one-stage oesophagectomy with oesophago-gastric anastomosis was performed, the management of carcinoma of the oesophagus continues to present many problems. Not least among these is the fact that the results of all current methods of treatment, with an overall five-year survival rate of about 5%, are so disappointing.

Oesophageal cancer is not a common disorder and it is therefore difficult for individual clinicians to acquire adequate experience regarding the many complex aspects of the disease and the most appropriate manner in which to manage it.

This report, based on The West Midlands Cancer Registry, seeks to remedy some of these deficiencies. Because of its ability to collect and collate data on 95% of all varieties of malignant disease occurring in a population of five million, the Registry has established an enviable international reputation in the epidemiological aspects of malignant disease and the results of its treatment.

I commend this study to its readers, for in the pages which follow they will find a great deal of authoritative facts which will stimulate their interest and improve our understanding of this dreaded disease. The work is both welcome and timely. I hope it will be the forerunner of many more of a similar nature, and I warmly congratulate all those who have worked so hard to bring it to fruition.

London WC2A 3PN, 1986   Sir Geoffrey Slaney, KBE
President
The Royal College of Surgeons of England

Acknowledgements

This book is based entirely on the data in the Birmingham and West Midlands Regional Cancer Registry.

We thank all those who — over many years — have given so generously of their time and expertise to ensure the completeness and accuracy of the data in the Registry. These include:

From hospitals:
Consultant clinicians and pathologists
Administrators
Junior medical staff
Laboratory technicians
Medical records staff
Medical secretaries

From the University of Birmingham:
The staff of the Computer Centre, Director Prof P. Jarratt

Throughout the Region:
Coroners
General practitioners
Staff of family practitioner committees

From the Registry:
All the staff (both past and present) and in particular Ms Claudia Roginski, the present Deputy Director, who was previously the statistician on the Monograph Team.

From the Monograph Team:
Mrs Vanessa Chadderton for her indefectible and indefatigable technical and secretarial help.

The Cancer Registry is supported mainly by the West Midlands Regional Health Authority.

The Monograph Project has been most generously supported by grants from:
Cancer Research Campaign
Department of Health and Social Security
Medical Research Council

1
Introduction and Methods

1.1 INTRODUCTION

Carcinoma of the oesophagus is a relatively uncommon tumour and reliable statistics about it are even less common. Since the organ lies in the neck, chest and abdomen, the tumours that it generates are dealt with by clinicians from many different disciplines, including otorhinolaryngologists, thoracic surgeons, general surgeons, gastro-enterologists, radiotherapists and oncologists. Consequently, not many acquire sufficient experience to form an accurate estimate of the nature and pattern of the disease. While the aetiology is largely unknown, it is clear that oesophageal carcinoma is increasing in incidence and is highly lethal.

It is these considerations which make this survey particularly important. The data presented here are based not on clinical series, but on information collected consistently by the Birmingham and West Midlands Cancer Registry from a large and stable population that is representative of the United Kingdom as a whole, over a recent 25-year period. The 95% efficiency rate of this registry, and the large number of cases surveyed, means that the results are both accurate and reliable in indicating the epidemiological, pathological and clinical trends that are occurring in this particular disease.

Recently, the problems of oesophageal carcinoma have begun to attract the scientific and clinical attention which they deserve. Investigations into the aetiology, oncogenesis and treatment of this tumour are being planned or undertaken, and the need for precise historical population data is correspondingly pressing. The aspects of the disease which have been chosen for analysis are those which are most likely to be of value to clinicians and epidemiologists, but it is clear that much additional information could be derived from the same material. In another publication based on these cases (British Journal of Surgery (1986), vol. 73, p. 621-3) we have demonstrated that the experience of the surgeon has a profound effect on the post-operative mortality and long-term survival following oesophageal resection for carcinoma, and this illustrates the way in which such

data can be used to identify and perhaps solve some of the un-
pleasant clinical and human problems associated with this malignancy.

1.2 INCLUSION CRITERIA

For this review, oesophageal carcinoma was defined as a malignant
tumour arising within the oesophagus itself, in accordance with
rubric 150 of the International Classification of Diseases (ICD, 1977).
Cases where the tumour was located at the extreme upper or lower
end of the oesophagus were individually reviewed; those which
appeared to arise in the hypopharynx were excluded and assigned to
a later survey of oral and pharyngeal tumours; carcinomas of the
cardia were similarly excluded and assigned to a survey of gastric
tumours. Classification according to site in the upper, middle or
lower third of the oesophagus was based on the description from the
reporting doctor, or information in the case records concerning the
radiological, endoscopic, operative or autopsy findings; cases in
which the precise site could not be identified are included as 'site
unspecified'.

In the majority of cases (69%) the diagnosis was based on
histological evidence obtained by cytology, biopsy, operation or
autopsy. Cases in which there was doubt as to whether the tumour
was malignant were individually reviewed, as were all adenocarcinomas of the lower oesophagus, the latter to determine whether
they should be considered as tumours arising primarily in the
stomach. Where histological evidence was not available (e.g. in
terminal cases) the diagnosis was based on radiological, endoscopic
or autopsy findings, or on the clinical course in the patient and the
certified cause of death. Further details of validation procedures
are given in Section 1.4.

1.3 DATA BASE

The results are based on the data in the Birmingham and West
Midlands Regional Cancer Registry (BRCR) which includes all new
cases of oesophageal carcinoma reported in the 25 years from 1957 to
1981 in the West Midlands. During this time there were no major
changes in the external boundaries of the Region and no alterations
in the methods of cancer registration. The Registry became population based in 1957 and by 1960 approximately 95% of all patients
were being registered (Waterhouse, 1974). A description of methods
of registration and a brief history of the Registry are given in
Appendix 1.

1.4 VALIDATION PROCEDURES

The essence of reliable statistics is accurate data. The precision of
the Registry's data base and the steps taken to enhance it are
discussed below.

Accuracy of the Raw Data

The accuracy of the original medical record could not be assessed as part of this study. However, at the next stage, i.e. transcription from hospital notes to Registry returns, the Registry is fortunate in having the active co-operation of radiotherapists throughout the region. As a result, in the main, either the original notes or photocopies are sent to the Registry for all patients seen at a Radiotherapy Centre. Details of those not treated by radiotherapy reach the Registry in a number of ways which have been in operation throughout the period of the survey (see Appendix 1). The Registry also receives copies of all pathology reports independently and these were invaluable in providing an independent audit, not only of histological type but also of nodal involvement and some aspects of surgical treatment.

Accuracy of Recording and Coding

The administrative data on age, date of birth, sex, anniversary date, date of death and survival is routinely validated at the time of input to the computer. In some instances this is by deliberate redundancy, for example, both age and date of birth are recorded.

The clinical material which forms a large part of the data base has always been coded at the Registry by trained nurses or their equivalent. These 'abstractors' have an intensive and continuing 'in-house' training and work in one room to ensure that differences of interpretation can readily be discussed. When a decision has been reached it is recorded in a manual of 'conventions' which each abstractor has, so that thereafter there is consistency of coding. The coded information is then subject to stringent quality-control checks which test, for instance, the compatibility of sex, site and histology.

In this study, routine computer checks were extended to cover as many of the parameters being analysed as possible. These validation procedures were time consuming to design, to program and to implement, but make the results far more accurate and reliable. They included reviewing the notes (which are kept in the Registry) for:

1. Cases where the sub-site was not specified.
2. Patients not treated curatively, but alive at 5 years or dying from causes other than cancer.
3. Patients without histological confirmation who survived 5 years.
4. Compatibility of histological type, source and site.
5. Compatibility of treatment policy (curative, palliative or exploratory) and operation code.

Additional information, particularly relating to histology and post-mortem results, was obtained for all doubtful cases, and we are indebted to the staff of pathology departments throughout the region for their ready response to requests for information on cases from many years ago.

1.5 SURVIVAL DATA

Five-year survival data is presented for 4680 patients registered in the 20-year period from 1957 to 1976. Of these, only six (0.13%) were lost to follow-up and only two of these had active treatment (radiotherapy); all were regarded as having died at the time of last follow-up.

Both crude and age-adjusted rates are given for overall survival, but thereafter age-adjusted rates are used for the reasons given below. In graphs, survival is expressed as a percentage of the starting population and survival is plotted monthly up to 1 year, two-monthly up to 2 years and then annually.

1.6 STATISTICAL METHODS

For the most part the numerical and graphical methods used will be self-evident to the reader, even if the subject in general is an unfamiliar one. Incidence rates by sex and age, for instance, are the quotients of the numbers of cases within a given sex and age group (e.g. females, aged 65-69) divided by the numbers of the population in the same sex and age group, although usually this quotient is expressed as a rate 'per hundred thousand', in order to provide a figure which is of a convenient size.

The scales of graphs may be linear, i.e. the scale numbers are evenly spaced (e.g. the space between the ages 60 and 70 is the same as that between 30 and 40). For many graphs, however, a logarithmic scale has been used, generally for the vertical measurement. In this, the space between the numbers 1 and 10 is the same as that between 10 and 100; or that between 2 and 4 is the same as that between 6 and 12. This makes it easier to encompass a very wide range of numbers (rates) and yet to be able to read them clearly, and means that slopes which are parallel will represent identical rates of change (e.g. an increase from 6 to 9 will be parallel to an increase from 40 to 60 if they each refer to an equivalent distance on the horizontal axis).

Another technique used in some of the graphs is that of 'moving averages'. It is a method frequently used to smooth some of the erratic swings of graphs that are based on small numbers. A two-point moving average begins with the average of the vertical scale readings of the first two points, plotted at a point on the horizontal scale midway between the readings for those two points. The next point on the graph is the average of the second and third points (again, for both scales), and after that the process continues in the same way. Each original point thus contributes to two of the points in the moving-average graph. It will be obvious that a

three-point moving average will consist of averages of three consecutive points, moving by successively dropping a point at one side
and adding the next point at the other side.

Crude rates, based on a simple numerator and denominator,
each being totals, can be misleading when used for purposes of
comparison. Incidence rates vary sharply with age, so that the
comparison of crude all-ages rates for populations with different age
structures can be very misleading. For the same reason, in comparing survival, it is necessary to adjust for the increase of general
mortality with age. To compensate for variations in age and sex,
age-standardised incidence rates (using the direct method) and
age-adjusted survival rates have been used throughout. This not
only enables the reader to relate the results to other series which
have been similarly adjusted for their age structure, but also
facilitates comparisons between subsets of these data. Details of
both methods are given in Appendix 2, which also quotes the 'World
Standard Population'; all standardised rates in the book have been
made to this population.

In all the numerical presentations of the data here analysed,
the actual numbers of cases are given in at least one of the tabu-
lations, so that full information is available to the reader. All tables
have been carefully cross-checked throughout, and to the best of
our knowledge they are both consistent and correct. We would like
to be informed of any errors that may be discovered.

We have also tabulated the census populations for the region
that we have used for various time periods. These we have obtained
from the census data published by HMSO for the Registrar General
and the OPCS (see References).

Tests of Statistical Significance

The tests of significance used are Student's t-test and the chi-
squared test (Bradford Hill, 1966). Where either of these tests of
statistical significance has been used to compare pairs of data, the
results have been indicated as:

Blank for either 'not significant' or not tested
* for $p < 0.05$ (the '5% level') = 'significant' in text
** for $p < 0.01$ (the '1% level') = 'highly significant'
*** for $p < 0.001$ (the '0.1% level') = 'very highly significant'

For example, in Table 3.3.2 the *** means that 10.5% has been
compared with 5.9% and found to be very highly significantly different ($p < 0.001$), and +++ means that the 22.4% was compared with
11.0%, with the same degree of significance.

1.7 POPULATION

The West Midlands (formerly the Birmingham) Region is fortunate in
not having suffered any changes in its external boundaries during
the period under review. The age and sex structure of the population is most accurately known at the time of the census. In
addition to published data, the OPCS have very kindly supplied
further information, both on revised estimates, particularly for
inter-censal years and on a more detailed breakdown for the older
ages.

In Figure 1.1 the two extreme populations in 1961 and 1981 are
compared. For each, the distributions - within each sex - have
been plotted for 5-year age groups. The resulting pyramid illustrates the ageing of the population observed in the last census, with
fewer individuals aged under 10 and more over 60. The somewhat
higher proportion of the 15-24-year groups in 1981 probably reflects
the high birth rates of the early 1960s.

The overall changes in the population in millions can be sum-
marised as follows:

Census year	Males	Females	Total	Changes(%)
1961	2.351	2.406	4.757 ⎫	
1971	2.528	2.582	5.110 ⎬	+7.4 ⎫ +7.2
1981	2.513	2.586	5.099 ⎭	−0.2 ⎭

A number of socio-economic factors, as identified in 1981, are
compared for the West Midlands and Great Britain in Table 1.1.
This shows that one of the major differences is in the higher proportion of people from the New Commonwealth and Pakistan, and the
smaller proportion from other countries outside the United Kingdom.
However, the proportionate change over the 10 years 1971 to 1981 is
less (5.9%) than for the country as a whole (8.9%), possibly indicating a reduction in the number of immigrants settling in this
region.

The industrial, urban and rural make-up of the region is
illustrated in Table 1.2. The West Midlands forms a tenth of the
population of England and Wales and, as can be seen, the socio-
economic structure and the varied industrial, urban and rural
pattern make it an ideal situation for the study of cancer, and its
representativeness also means that the results can be applied not
only to other regions but also to other countries.

A number of different time periods are used in the book and
Table 1.3 gives the populations used as the denominator for each
time period. Details of the age and sex structure of each population
are given in Appendix 3.

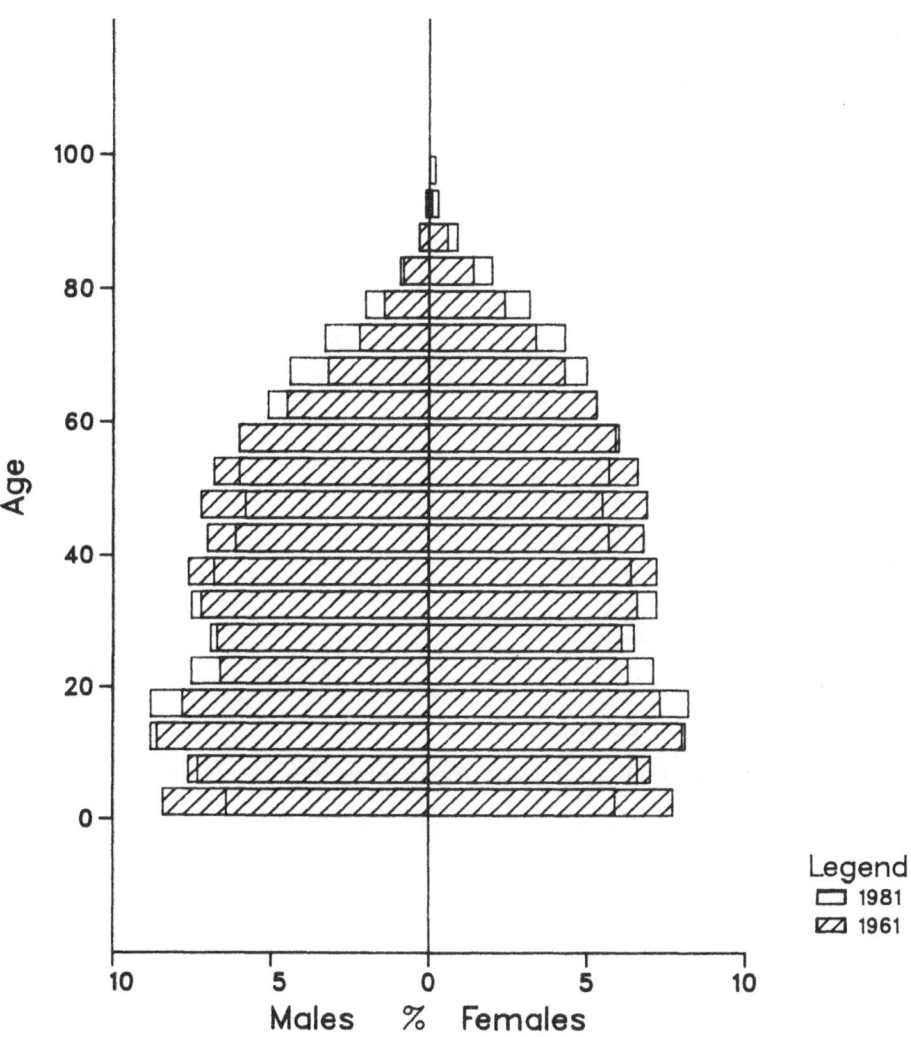

Figure 1.1   1961 and 1981 Census Population Pyramid.

Table 1.1 Comparison of Social Factors, in 1981, for West Midlands Region and Great Britain.

	West Midlands Region	Great Britain
Country of Birth		
Percentage of population born in:		
Irish Republic	1.5	1.1
New Commonwealth & Pakistan	3.8	2.8
Other countries outside U.K.	1.3	2.3
1971–81 change (%) in number born outside U.K.	5.9	8.9
Social class (10% sample)		
Percentage of population in households with heads in Social Class:		
I	3.8	4.5
II	17.4	18.8
III Non-maual	7.8	9.1
Manual	29.4	26.2
IV	14.2	12.2
V	3.9	4.1
Armed forces or inadequately described	2.3	2.4
Head economically inactive +	21.2	22.7

+ Only economically active heads of households have been assigned a social class.

Higher Education (10% sample)		
Percentage of population * with higher education qualifications		
Men	12.2	13.7
Women	10.4	12.2

* 16 or over and in employment.

Taken from 'Key statistics for Local Authorities, Great Britain Census 1981'.

Table 1.2   Population Densities.

Family		Cluster		Proportion of West Midlands Population (%)
1A	Established high status areas	2	Suburban areas	
			North Birmingham	3.2
			Rugby	1.7
			Solihull	3.8
			South Warwickshire	4.2
1B	Higher status growth areas	5	Larger, more urbanised growth areas	
			Bromsgrove & Redditch	3.0
			Mid-Staffordshire	5.8
			South East Staffordshire	4.8
2A	More rural areas	8	Remoter rural areas	
			Herefordshire	2.9
		9	Less remote, mainly rural areas	
			Worcester and District	4.5
3	Mixed town and country, areas with some industry	11	More rural areas with industry	
			Kidderminster & District	1.9
			Shropshire	7.3
		13	More industrial areas	
			Dudley	5.8
			North Staffordshire	9.0
			North Warwickshire	3.4
			Walsall	5.2
4A	Traditional manufacturing areas	15	The Black country and similar	
			Central Birmingham	3.6
			East Birmingham	3.9
			Sandwell	6.0
			West Birmingham	4.0
			Wolverhampton	4.9
		16	Pennine towns and similar	
			Coventry	6.2
4B	Service centres and cities	17	Cities and more industrial service areas	
			South Birmingham	4.9
				100.0

Table 1.3   Populations Used for the Different Time Periods.

Time period	Population used
Quinquennium	
1957–61	1961
1962–66	1966
1967–71	1971
1972–76	1976
1977–81	1981
Decade	
1957–66	1961
1967–76	1971
1962–71	1966
1972–81	1976
Twenty five years	
1957–81	1971

1.8   GENERAL ARRANGEMENT

All tumours (except three primary lymphomas), whether carcinoma or of some other histology, are included in the analysis up to Table 3.2.   The 25 malignant but non-carcinomatous tumours are then excluded from the subsequent analyses and are described separately in Chapter 7, with the three lymphomas.   In the *Contents* section each individual set of data is listed and numbered separately; this numbering is used for cross-reference throughout the work and serves instead of an index.   Figures which relate to tabular data are given the same number as the relevant table and are placed on facing pages whenever possible.   All individual data is annotated as appropriate.   Methods which are relevant only to specific chapters are described in the brief introduction to each chapter.

2

Epidemiology: Demographic Aspects

Between 1957 and 1981, 6398 patients were registered with oeso-phageal tumours of all histological types, excluding only three primary lymphomas of the oesophagus which are considered separately in Chapter 7; this is to conform to the ICD definition of rubric 150.

This chapter presents the demographic aspects of the disease, by relating the cases to the populations from which they arose (see Chapter 1). Both numbers and rates are given, and for the examination of trends the overall period of 25 years has been subdivided into five groups of five consecutive years (quinquennia).

To allow for the changes by age in the structure of the population of the region over the quarter century, and also to render the results comparable with those from other centres, several of the rates have been presented in age-standardised (or age-adjusted) form. The methods used are given in Appendix 2.

All incidence rates are calculated 'per 100 000' and refer to a base of 1 year; where they are calculated for a period of 5 years, for instance, the overall rate is divided by five, to yield an *average annual rate*. To save unnecessary complexity, the headings to tables quote 'incidence rates', but they are in fact average annual rates, whatever the period of time that may be used in the table. In the figures all the incidence rates have been set against a logarithmic vertical scale, for the reasons given in Chapter 1.

2.1 SUMMARY OF FINDINGS

For the whole period, the crude rate was 5.01 tumours per 100 000 population and the age-standardised rate was 3.31.

The rising number of patients of both sexes over the quarter century, seen best in Figure 2.1, is the result of at least three influences - firstly, for the initial 3 years, a steady improvement in the registration efficiency, which attained about 95% by 1960; secondly, the effect of ageing of the population (i.e. the increasing numbers in the older age groups, where the incidence of the disease increases rapidly); and thirdly, an increase in the incidence of the disease itself (see also Chapter 3).

It is the middle and lower thirds, in both sexes, which have shown a steady increase during the whole period (Figure 2.4). This increase is analysed further with respect to histological cell type in Chapter 3. The upper third has remained nearly stable in males and has shown a slight decrease in females.

Dividing both population and cases into groups (cohorts) according to their birth-years (Figure 2.13) shows a tendency in both sexes for the more recently born to have higher incidence rates. This implies that the risk in younger people is greater at each age than it was for their elders when they were at the same age.

The trend in the number of cases (Table 2.1), in conjunction with the fact that two thirds are over the age of 65 (Table 2.7), stresses the increasing clinical workload they represent, as well as their needs for general social and health care.

Table 2.1

This table shows a considerable rise in the number of cases, of both sexes, over the 25 years.   In the quinquennium from 1962-1966 there were 1175 cases compared with 1696 cases in 1977-1981; this represents an increase of 44% at a time when the population of the region increased by only 7.2% and registration was 95% complete. Later analysis indicates that this rise is due partly to increasing numbers in the older age groups in the population (where the incidence of the disease increases rapidly), and partly to an increase in the incidence of the disease itself.   There is also a steady decline in the male/female ratio which is further analysed in Chapter 3.

Table 2.1   All Tumours: Number of New Patients per Annum, 1957-81.

Year	Number of patients				Total in quinquennium	Sex ratio M/F
	Male	Female	Total			
1957	74	48	122			
1958	93	57	150			
1959	110	86	196		864	1.39 : 1
1960	107	82	189			
1961	118	89	207			
1962	131	95	226			
1963	148	106	254			
1964	122	95	217		1175	1.30 : 1
1965	131	105	236			
1966	133	109	242			
1967	129	100	229			
1968	139	98	237			
1969	124	128	252		1214	1.20 : 1
1970	140	118	258			
1971	131	107	238			
1972	165	116	281			
1973	144	131	275			
1974	153	116	269		1449	1.24 : 1
1975	163	131	294			
1976	176	154	330			
1977	189	158	347			
1978	187	147	334			
1979	172	148	320		1696	1.19 : 1
1980	185	168	353			
1981	190	152	342			
1957 - 81	3554	2844	6398			1.25 : 1

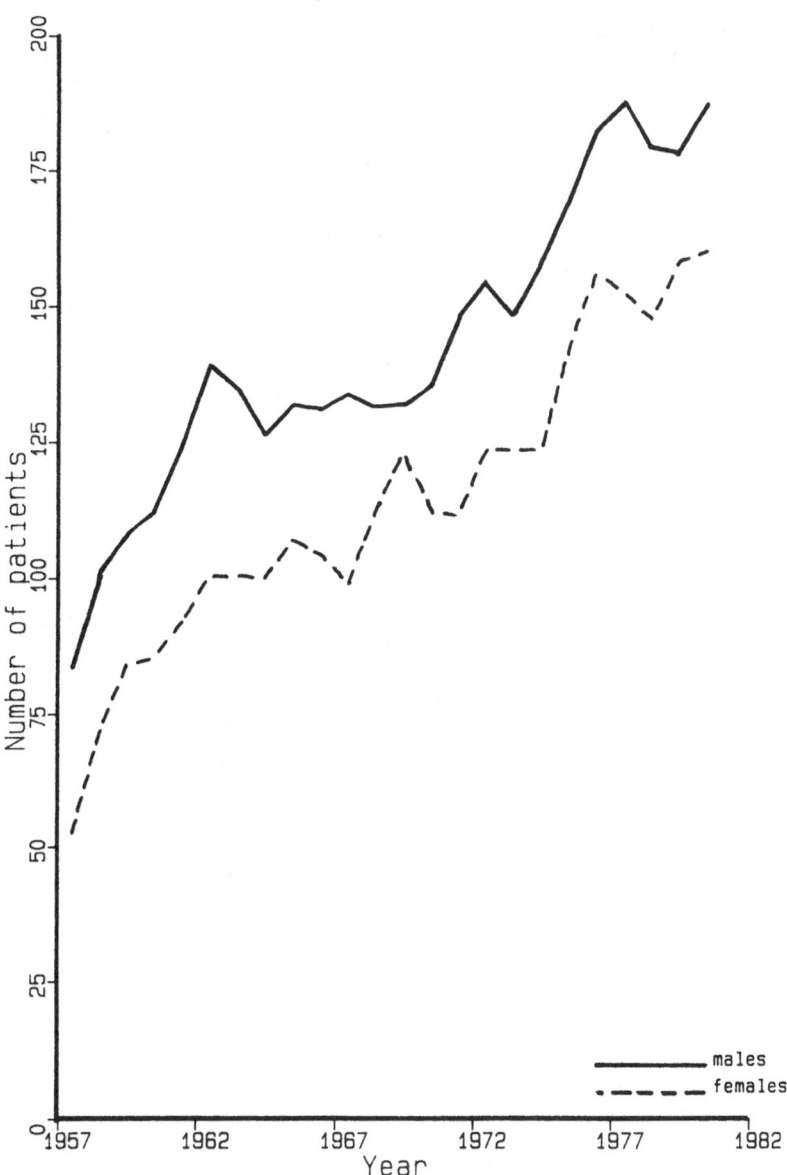

Figure 2.1   All Tumours: Number per Annum by Sex, 1957–81.
(Two-point moving average)

Table 2.2

Age-standardised incidence rates show that the disease is commoner
in males than in females. Over the 25 years, both sexes have shown
an increase in incidence, but in percentage terms this is greater for
females than for males, being 28% compared with 15% in the last 20
years when the efficiency of registration was relatively constant.
The incidence in females has shown a steady rise, but for males
there was a trough for the period 1967-1971; this was due to a drop
in the numbers of male cases and not to a change in the population.

Table 2.2   Average Annual Incidence Rates by Quinquennium and
            Sex.

Years	Crude incidence rates			Age standardised incidence rates		
	Males	Females	Combined	Males	Females	Combined
1957–61	4.27	3.01	3.63	3.58	1.90	2.59
1962–66	5.45	4.09	4.76	4.44	2.45	3.24
1967–71	5.25	4.27	4.75	4.11	2.49	3.13
1972–76	6.27	4.94	5.60	4.58	2.71	3.49
1977–81	7.35	5.98	6.65	5.09	3.13	3.98
1957–81	5.62	4.41	5.01	4.41	2.56	3.31

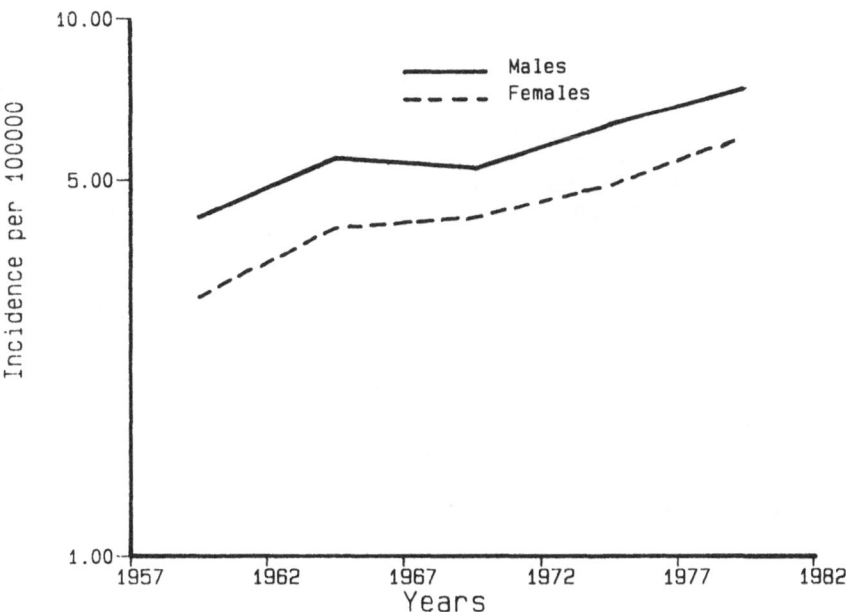

Figure 2.2.1   Incidence Rates by Quinquennium and Sex (crude).

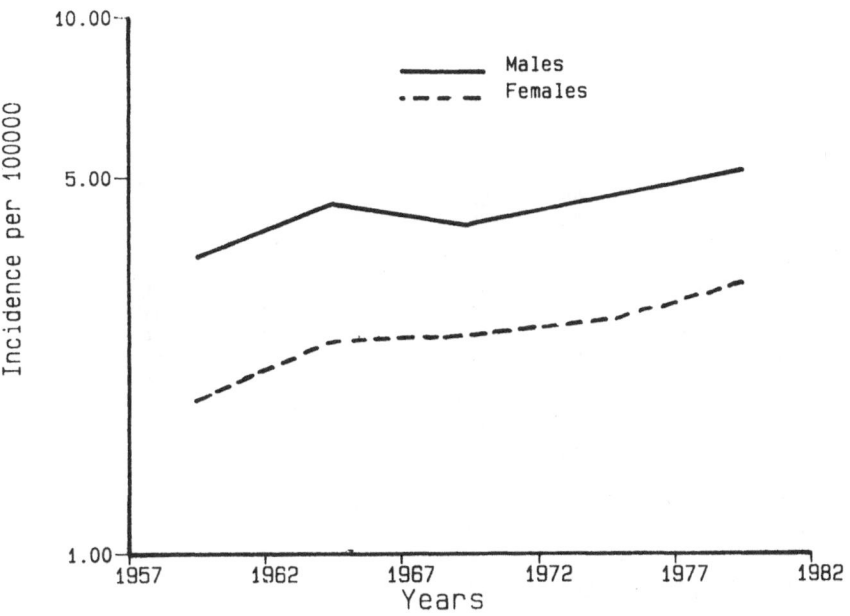

Figure 2.2.2   Incidence Rates by Quinquennium and Sex (age adjusted

Clinical Cancer Monographs: Oesophagus

Table 2.3

Clearly, the increasing number of cases is due mainly to an increase
in the number of tumours in the middle and lower thirds of the
oesophagus, which has almost amounted to a doubling in the period
under review. In the upper third and site unspecified groups there
has been no systematic change - particularly if the early years
(when registration was less complete) are excluded. In the lower
third, male cases always exceed female cases by some 30-40%, but in
all the other groups there is only a slight male excess, often with a
crossing over.

Table 2.3   Numbers per Annum by Site and Sex.

Year	Upper third male	Upper third female	Middle third male	Middle third female	Lower third male	Lower third female	Site unspecified male	Site unspecified female
1957	6	6	18	15	24	16	26	11
1958	8	6	17	8	50	37	18	6
1959	8	15	46	33	32	23	24	15
1960	6	8	50	28	33	28	18	18
1961	9	9	38	36	52	28	19	16
1962	18	15	40	24	52	36	21	20
1963	18	14	41	43	67	35	22	14
1964	15	8	35	27	58	48	14	12
1965	15	15	42	36	54	44	20	10
1966	13	9	44	45	62	35	14	20
1967	11	8	47	42	54	41	17	9
1968	16	10	53	37	52	43	18	8
1969	12	15	44	52	59	49	9	12
1970	16	10	43	46	71	53	10	9
1971	14	8	53	41	55	53	9	5
1972	16	11	61	45	73	53	15	7
1973	6	14	57	61	64	39	17	17
1974	13	14	60	49	66	44	14	9
1975	10	9	61	52	72	47	20	23
1976	11	16	75	57	77	56	13	25
1977	16	8	74	70	85	67	14	13
1978	14	14	74	75	85	50	14	8
1979	19	9	57	67	86	56	10	16
1980	12	9	67	63	87	79	19	17
1981	14	12	67	63	89	54	20	23
1957–81	316	272	1264	1115	1559	1114	415	343

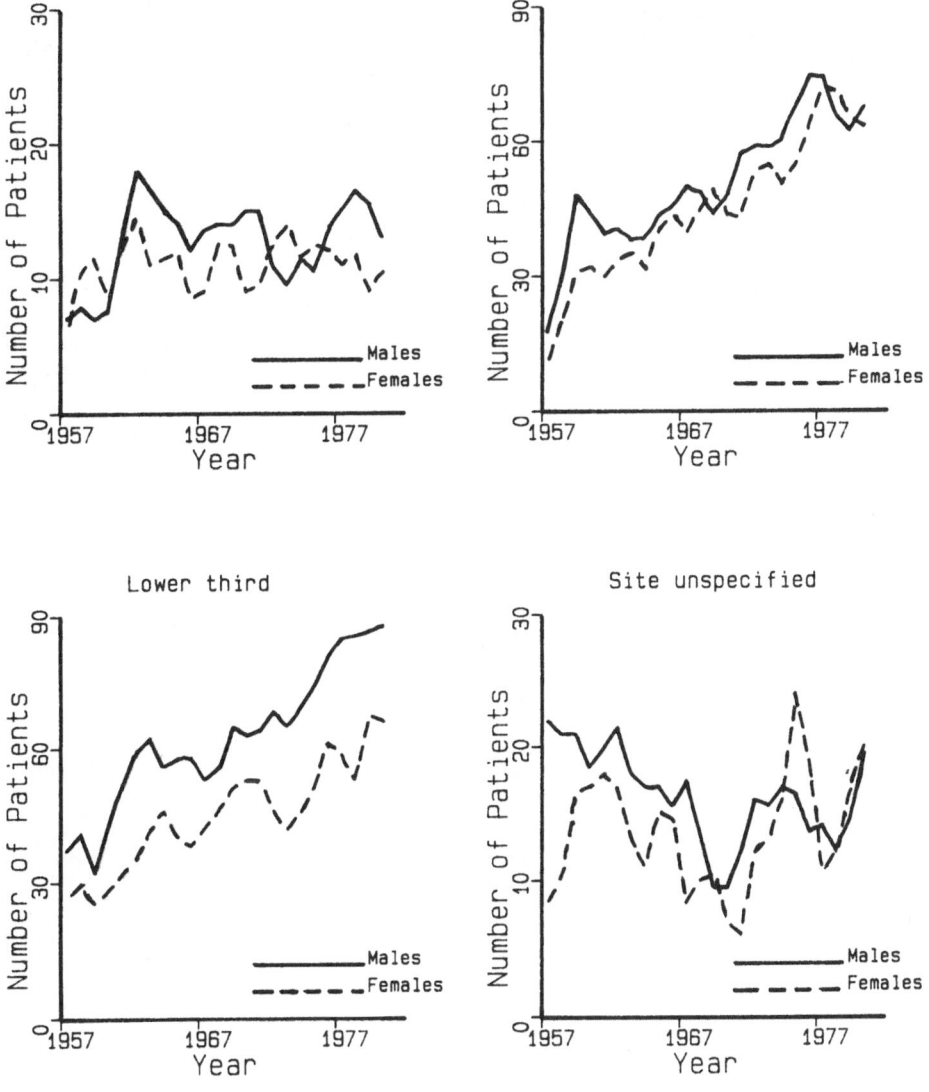

Figure 2.3   Numbers per Annum by Site and Sex.
(Two-point moving average)

Table 2.4

These age-standardised incidence rates show much the same trend as
in Section 2.3. The fact that the upper-third and site-unspecified
groups have remained substantially unchanged, while the middle- and
lower-third groups have increased, suggests that this rise represents a true increase in incidence in these parts of the oesophagus, and not merely a change in the classification. There is
little difference in behaviour between the sexes, except for the
consistent excess for males with lower-third tumours, as already
noted. The increased incidence in middle-third tumours is significant in females.

Table 2.4   Age Standardised Incidence Rates by Quinquennium, Site
            and Sex.

| Years | Upper third | | Middle third | | Lower third | | Site unspecified | |
	Male	Female	Male	Female	Male	Female	Male	Female
1957–61	0.26	0.25	1.19	0.64	1.36	0.70	0.78	0.32
1962–66	0.53	0.31	1.35	0.88*	1.93	0.95	0.63	0.32
1967–71	0.44	0.23	1.46	1.01	1.79	1.06	0.43	0.18
1972–76	0.31	0.28	1.77	1.18	2.05	0.94	0.45	0.31
1977–81	0.41	0.23	1.85	1.43*	2.40	1.22	0.44	0.26

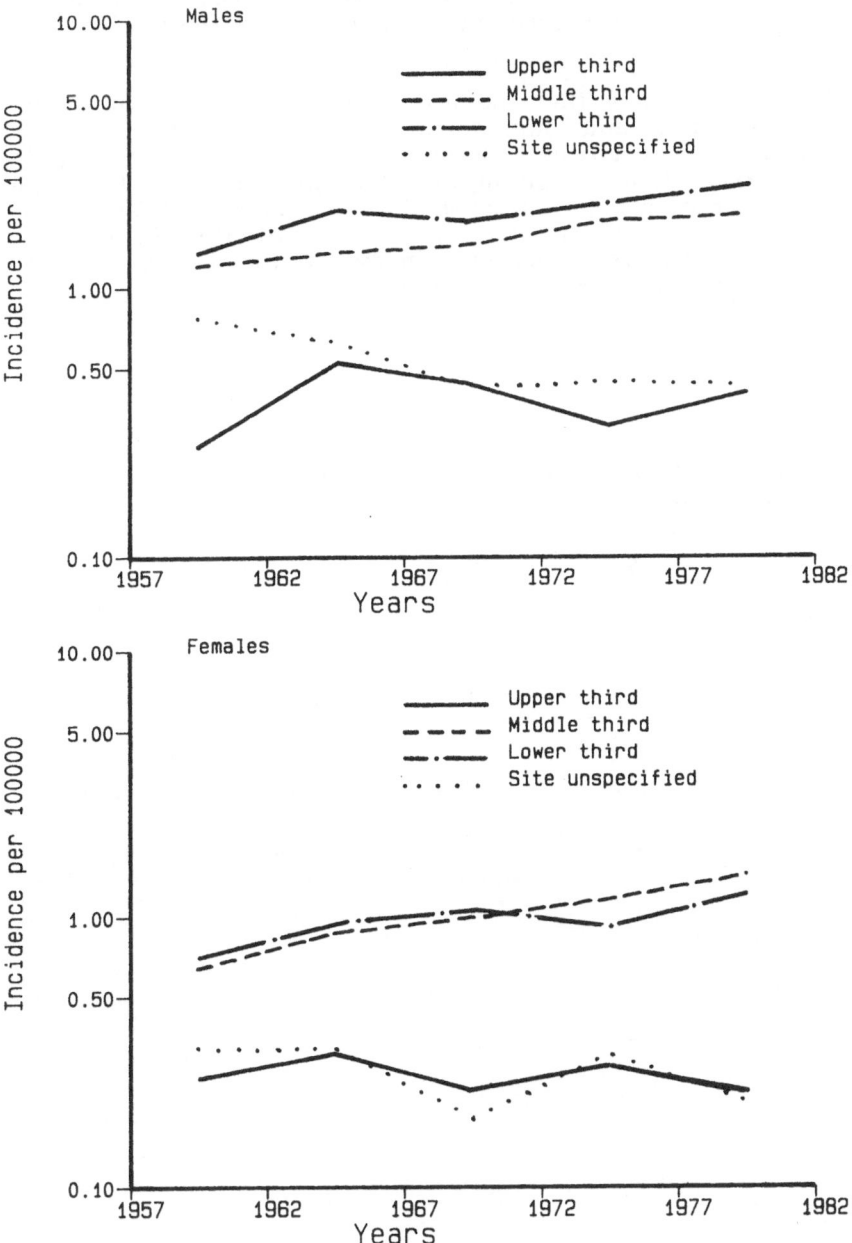

Figure 2.4 Incidence Rates by Quinquennium, Site and Sex.

Table 2.5

Each distribution has been calculated as a proportion of the total with known site, since it cannot be assumed that tumours included in 'site unspecified' have the same site distribution as those where the site is known.

This data indicates that the majority of tumours occur almost equally in the middle and lower thirds of the oesophagus. As the number of these has increased there has inevitably been a drop in the percentage of tumours arising in the upper third. The high proportion of middle-third tumours in this survey (42%) is at variance with many clinical series, but should reflect the true distribution of tumours within the body of the oesophagus, as tumours of the cardia have been excluded.

Table 2.5   Site Distribution (%) by Quinquennium (excluding site unspecified).

Quinquennium	Upper	Middle	Lower	
1957–61	11.7	41.7	46.6	100.0
1962–66	13.9	37.4	48.7	100.0
1967–71	10.8	41.3	47.9	100.0
1972–76	9.3	44.8	45.9	100.0
1977–81	8.2	43.9	47.9	100.0
1957–81	10.4	42.2	47.4	100.0

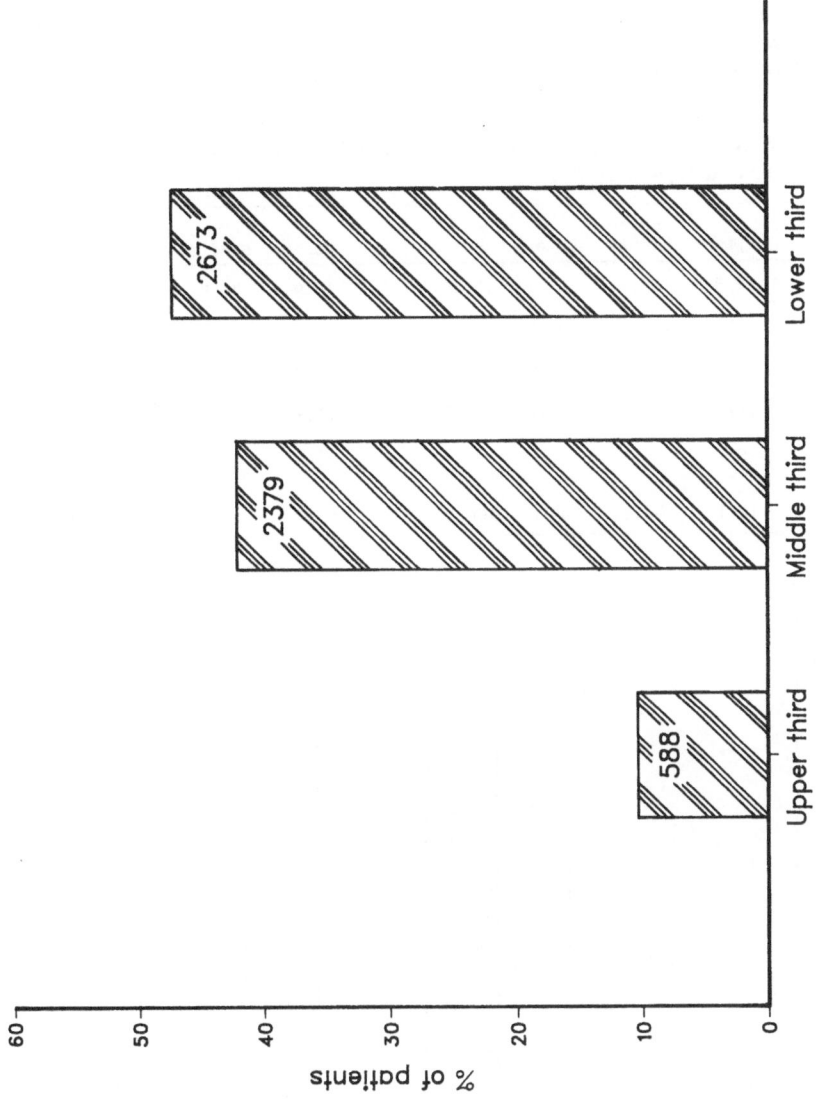

Figure 2.5 Distribution by Known Site, 1957–81.

Table 2.6

This data for the whole 25 years shows that there is no substantial difference in the sex distribution of tumours within the three main sites in the body of the oesophagus (Figure 2.6.1).

The analysis of each quinquennium within the 25 years shows a crossing over in females, with middle-third tumours exceeding those in the lower third from 1972 onwards; there is no comparable change with respect to males (Figure 2.6.2).

Table 2.6 Site Distribution (%) by Quinquennium and Sex (excluding site unspecified).

Quinquennium	Upper	Male Middle	Lower		Upper	Female Middle	Lower	
1957–61	9.3	42.6	48.1	100.0	14.9	40.5	44.6	100.0
1962–66	13.8	35.2	51.0	100.0	14.1	40.3	45.6	100.0
1967–71	11.5	40.0	48.5	100.0	10.0	42.9	47.1	100.0
1972–76	7.8	43.5	48.7	100.0	11.3	46.6	42.1	100.0
1977–81	8.9	40.1	51.0	100.0	7.5	48.5	44.0	100.0
1977–81	10.1	40.3	49.6	100.0	10.9	44.6	44.5	100.0

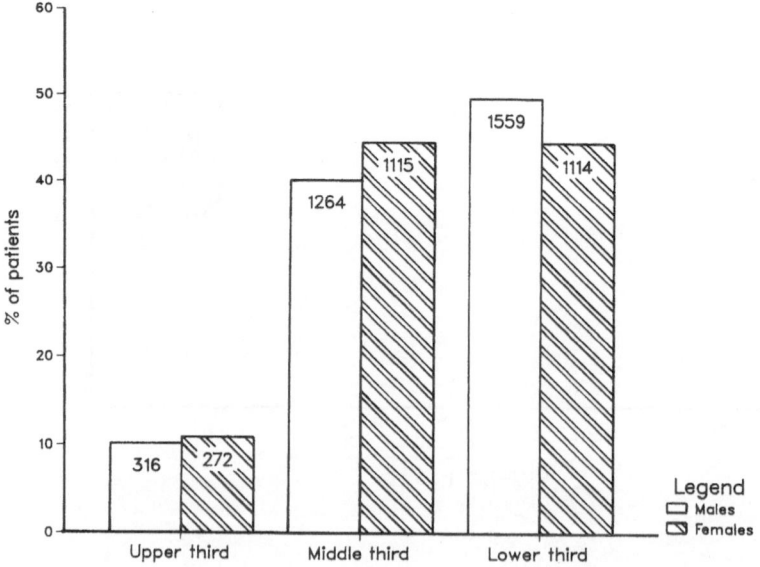

Figure 2.6.1 Site Distribution by Sex, 1957–81.

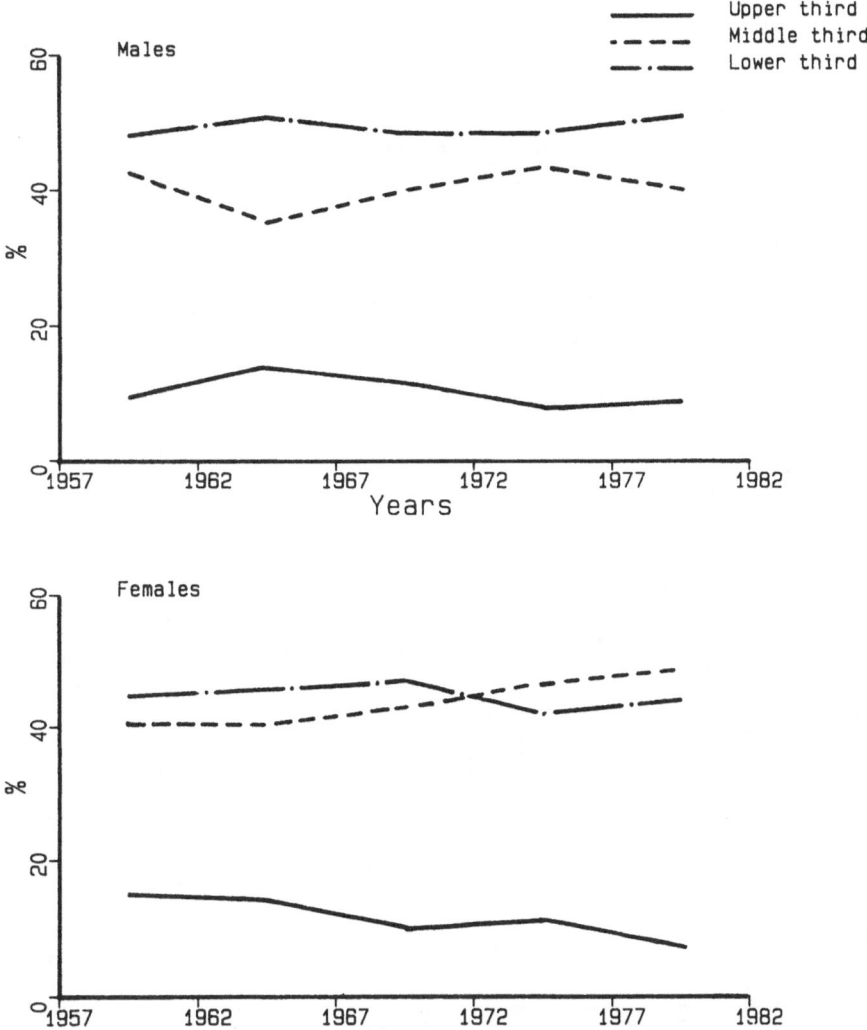

Figure 2.6.2 Site Distribution by Quinquennium and Sex.

Table 2.7

Results in this section represent averages for the whole period and show little difference between the sexes until about the age of 50, when the incidence for males begins to exceed that for females.   As the data covers a long period of time during which there have been numerous variations, it is subdivided for further analysis in Section 2.10 onwards.

Table 2.7   Numbers and Incidence Rates by Age and Sex, 1957-81 (All sites).

Age group	Number of patients			Incidence rate per 100,000		
	Male	Female	Total	Male	Female	Total
0 – 19	0	0	0	-	-	-
20 – 24	1	1	2	0.02	0.02	0.02
25 – 29	3	0	3	0.07	0.00	0.03
30 – 34	6	12	18	0.15	0.32	0.23
35 – 39	20	16	36	0.52	0.44	0.48
40 – 44	44	50	94	1.08	1.28	1.18
45 – 49	118	108	226	2.79	2.59	2.69
50 – 54	235	194	429	6.13	5.01	5.56
55 – 59	400	268	668	10.63	7.05	8.83
60 – 64	529	336	865	16.15	9.45	12.66
65 – 69	654	394	1048	25.84	12.89	18.76
70 – 74	615	456	1071	39.34	18.65	26.72
75 – 79	502	440	942	56.38	25.86	36.35
80 – 84	279	334	613	61.07	32.29	41.11
85 – 89	113	174	287	65.22	37.07	44.66
90 – 94	30	52	82	67.04	37.14	44.38
95+	4	9	13	58.18	33.96	38.95
Unknown	1	0	1			
All ages	3554	2844	6398	5.62	4.41	5.01

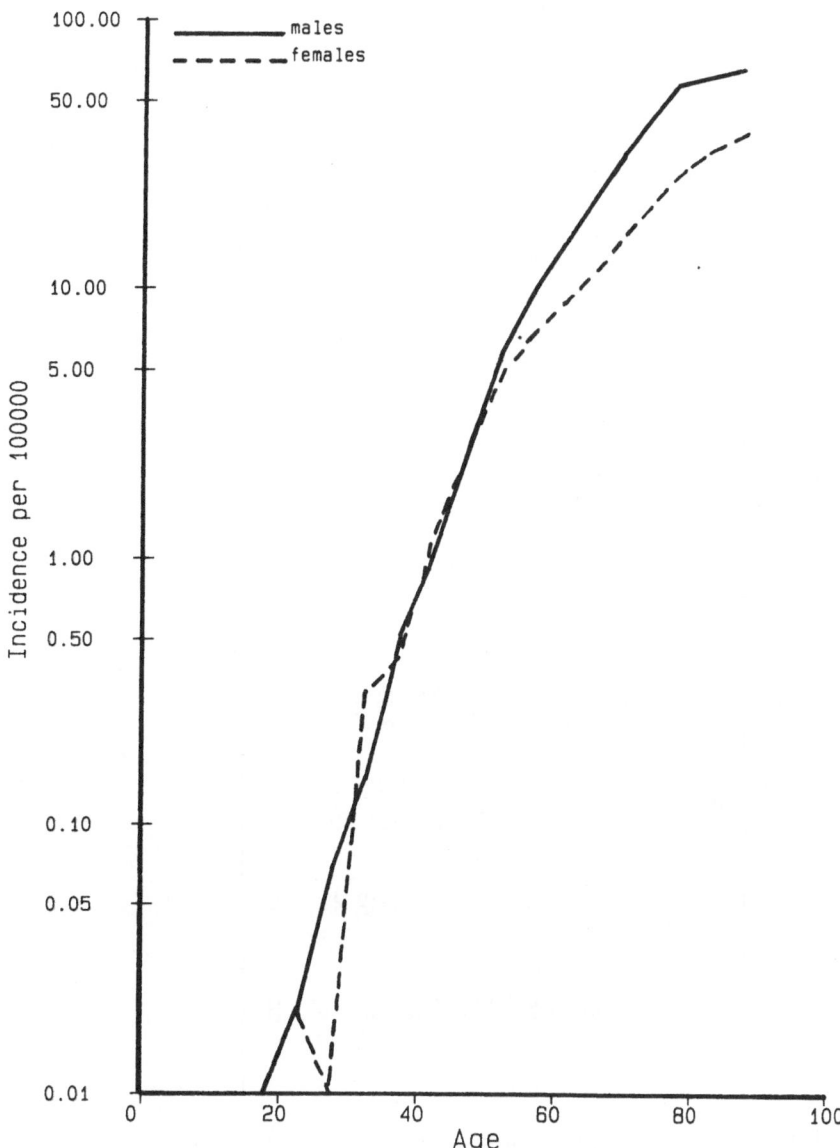

Figure 2.7   Incidence Rates by Age and Sex, 1957–81.

Table 2.8

The increased incidence with age is shown here to apply to all subsites and both sexes, and all four graphs are similar in their slope and general form.

Table 2.8 Incidence Rates by Age, Site and Sex, 1957-81.

Age group	Upper third		Middle third		Lower third		Site unspecified	
	Male	Female	Male	Female	Male	Female	Male	Female
0 – 19	–	–	–	–	–	–	–	–
20 – 24	0.02	–	–	0.02	–	–	–	–
25 – 29	0.02	–	0.02	–	0.02	–	–	–
30 – 34	–	0.03	0.03	0.26	0.12	0.03	–	–
35 – 39	0.13	0.14	0.10	0.19	0.26	0.11	0.03	–
40 – 45	0.15	0.23	0.44	0.51	0.42	0.44	0.07	0.10
45 – 49	0.17	0.31	0.88	1.08	1.54	1.06	0.21	0.14
50 – 54	0.70	0.36	2.40	2.45	2.58	2.01	0.44	0.18
55 – 59	1.12	1.00	4.01	2.84	4.76	2.94	0.74	0.26
60 – 64	1.16	0.79	6.23	4.30	7.51	3.49	1.25	0.87
65 – 69	2.13	1.47	9.96	5.53	11.34	4.81	2.41	1.08
70 – 74	3.58	1.76	13.69	7.49	16.95	7.04	5.12	2.37
75 – 79	4.27	1.76	19.32	9.46	23.81	11.23	8.99	3.41
80 – 84	6.35	2.22	18.61	9.96	25.61	14.41	10.51	5.70
85 – 89	6.35	2.98	15.58	9.16	24.24	13.00	19.05	11.93
90 – 94	–	5.00	13.41	10.71	26.82	9.29	26.82	12.14
95+	14.55	7.55	–	7.55	29.09	3.77	14.55	15.09
All ages	0.50	0.42	2.00	1.73	2.47	1.73	0.66	0.53

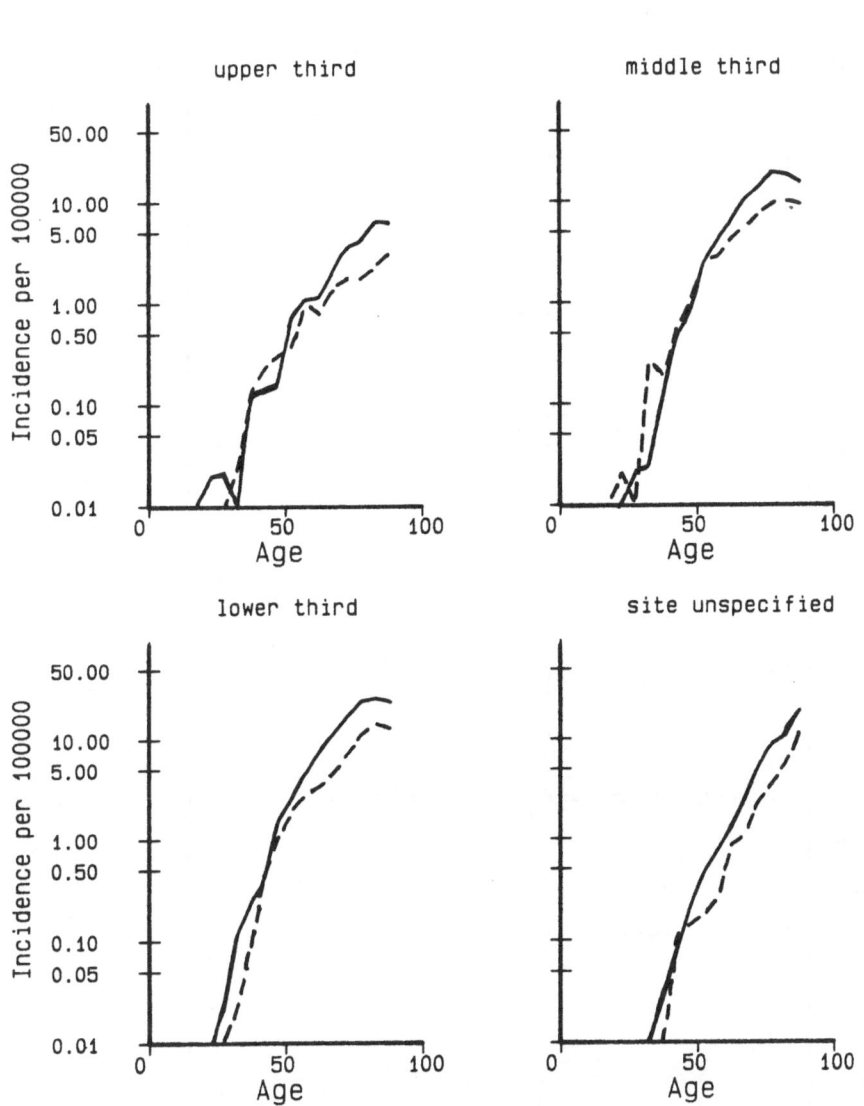

Figure 2.8   Incidence Rates by Age, Site and Sex, 1957-81.

Table 2.9

This table provides the raw data for Table 2.8. It is given to enable the reader to calculate different age groupings, if desired.

Table 2.9 Numbers by Age, Site and Sex, 1957-81.

Age group	Upper third Male	Upper third Female	Middle third Male	Middle third Female	Lower third Male	Lower third Female	Site unspecified Male	Site unspecified Female
0 – 19	0	0	0	0	0	0	0	0
20 – 24	1	0	0	1	0	0	0	0
25 – 29	1	0	1	0	1	0	0	0
30 – 34	0	1	1	10	5	1	0	0
35 – 39	5	5	4	7	10	4	1	0
40 – 44	6	9	18	20	17	17	3	4
45 – 49	7	13	37	45	65	44	9	6
50 – 54	27	14	92	95	99	78	17	7
55 – 59	42	38	151	108	179	112	28	10
60 – 64	38	28	204	153	246	124	41	31
65 – 69	54	45	252	169	287	147	61	33
70 – 74	56	43	214	183	265	172	80	58
75 – 79	38	30	172	161	212	191	80	58
80 – 84	29	23	85	103	117	149	48	59
85 – 89	11	14	27	43	42	61	33	56
90 – 94	0	7	6	15	12	13	12	17
95+	1	2	0	2	2	1	1	4
Unknown	0	0	0	0	0	0	1	0
All ages	316	272	1264	1115	1559	1114	415	343

Table 2.10

This table gives numbers by sex and age for each quinquennium. The reader can therefore calculate different groupings (e.g. 1957-1966), if desired.

Table 2.10   Numbers by Age, Quinquennium and Sex.

Age group	1957 - 61 Male	1957 - 61 Female	1962 - 66 Male	1962 - 66 Female	1967 - 71 Male	1967 - 71 Female	1972 - 76 Male	1972 - 76 Female	1977 - 81 Male	1977 - 81 Female
0 - 19	0	0	0	0	0	0	0	0	0	0
20 - 24	0	0	1	0	0	0	0	0	0	1
25 - 29	1	0	1	0	0	0	0	0	1	0
30 - 34	2	2	0	3	1	3	3	2	0	2
35 - 39	5	4	5	2	2	3	3	4	5	3
40 - 44	6	6	8	12	11	14	7	9	12	9
45 - 49	18	14	24	35	25	29	23	18	28	12
50 - 54	33	34	39	21	46	38	57	48	60	53
55 - 59	62	27	77	49	73	62	87	62	101	68
60 - 64	63	49	103	58	104	57	136	73	123	99
65 - 69	103	57	99	74	109	64	148	93	195	106
70 - 74	87	66	116	80	117	92	138	110	157	108
75 - 79	69	47	102	72	90	86	108	96	133	139
80 - 84	36	38	55	62	58	69	58	72	72	93
85 - 89	14	13	30	32	19	28	26	46	24	55
90 - 94	3	4	5	10	7	5	6	14	9	19
95+	0	1	0	0	1	1	1	1	2	6
Unknown	0	0	0	0	0	0	0	0	1	0
All ages	502	362	665	510	663	551	801	648	923	773

Table 2.11

Figures for all sites have been combined into decades to increase their stability. There is a striking similarity in the pattern of rising incidence with age in both sexes over the two decades. In both sexes there is a slight increase in the second decade, as noted previously, but it is more consistent at each age in males.

Table 2.11 Incidence Rates by Age, Decade and Sex.

Age group	1962 – 71 Male	1962 – 71 Female	1972 – 81 Male	1972 – 81 Female
0 – 19	–	–	–	0.06
20 – 24	0.06	–	–	–
25 – 29	0.06	–	0.05	–
30 – 34	0.06	0.39	0.17	0.24
35 – 39	0.42	0.31	0.51	0.47
40 – 44	1.16	1.63	1.25	1.24
45 – 49	2.89	3.85	3.24	1.97
50 – 54	5.41	3.75	7.23	6.25
55 – 59	10.32	7.49	12.86	8.63
60 – 64	17.50	8.56	19.29	11.88
65 – 69	23.68	12.23	31.01	15.16
70 – 74	40.43	19.25	38.51	20.22
75 – 79	55.72	25.10	58.64	30.56
80 – 84	62.66	34.96	67.01	36.18
85 – 89	74.32	37.33	69.44	46.98
90 – 95	83.51	34.70	78.95	46.48
95+	50.25	12.67	75.00	41.18
All ages	5.44	4.25	6.74	5.42

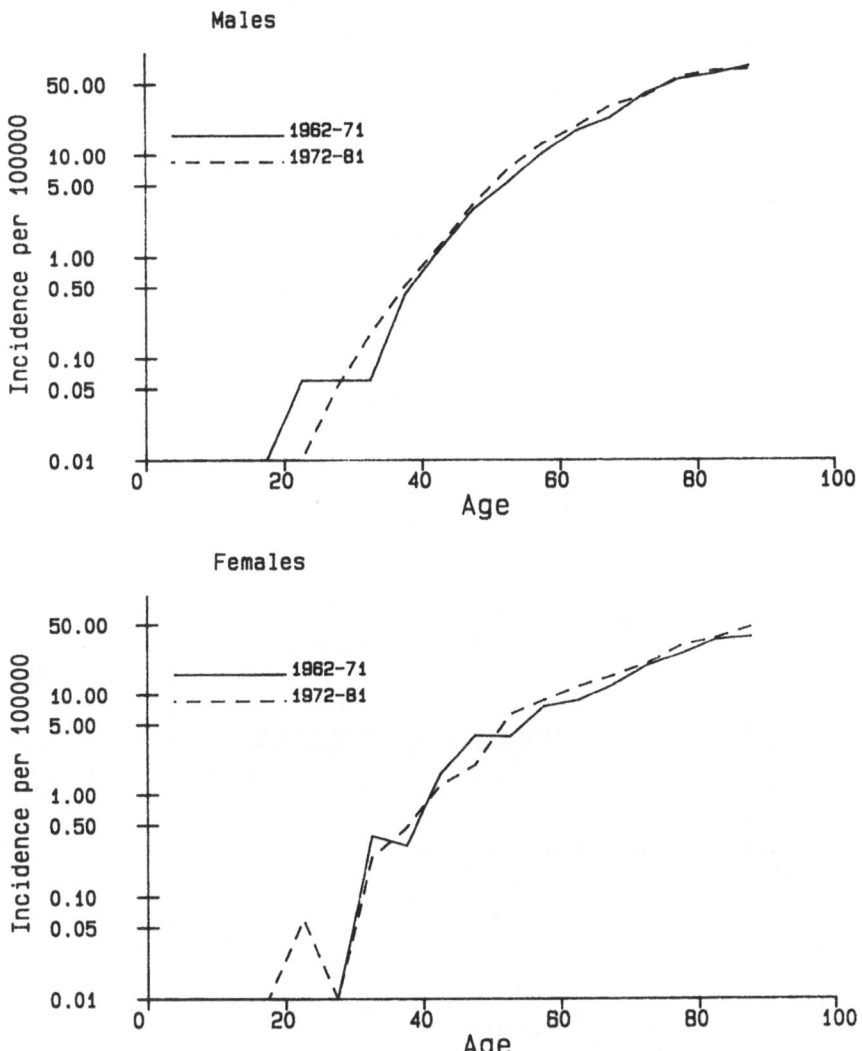

Figure 2.11   Incidence Rates by Age, Decade and Sex.

Table 2.12

The quinquennial figures of Table 2.10 have been put together into decades, as for all sites, to increase their stability. As with Table 2.11 they show a close similarity within each subsite.

Table 2.12.1   Incidence Rates by Age, Site and Sex. Decade 1962–71.

Age group	Upper third Male	Upper third Female	Middle third Male	Middle third Female	Lower third Male	Lower third Female	Site unspecified Male	Site unspecified Female
0 – 19	–	–	–	–	–	–	–	–
20 – 24	0.06	–	–	–	–	–	–	–
25 – 29	0.06	–	–	–	–	–	–	–
30 – 34	–	0.07	–	0.26	0.06	0.07	–	–
35 – 39	0.12	0.06	0.12	0.13	0.18	0.13	–	–
40 – 44	0.24	0.31	0.18	0.69	0.67	0.50	0.06	0.13
45 – 49	0.18	0.48	1.36	1.51	1.06	1.57	0.30	0.30
50 – 54	0.76	0.26	2.10	1.91	2.10	1.53	0.45	0.06
55 – 59	1.31	0.95	3.23	2.63	5.50	3.58	0.28	0.34
60 – 64	1.69	1.04	6.93	3.43	7.44	3.35	1.44	0.75
65 – 69	2.28	0.80	7.63	5.23	11.73	5.58	2.05	0.62
70 – 74	3.64	2.46	14.23	7.61	17.18	7.27	5.38	1.90
75 – 79	6.38	1.91	17.70	9.69	22.34	10.64	9.29	2.86
80 – 84	7.21	2.94	16.63	8.54	27.72	16.55	11.09	6.94
85 – 89	13.65	3.73	15.17	7.47	24.27	11.20	21.24	14.93
90 – 94	–	9.25	13.92	9.25	34.80	6.94	34.80	9.25
95+	50.25	12.67	–	–	–	–	–	–
All ages	0.61	0.45	1.81	1.58	2.39	1.75	0.63	0.48

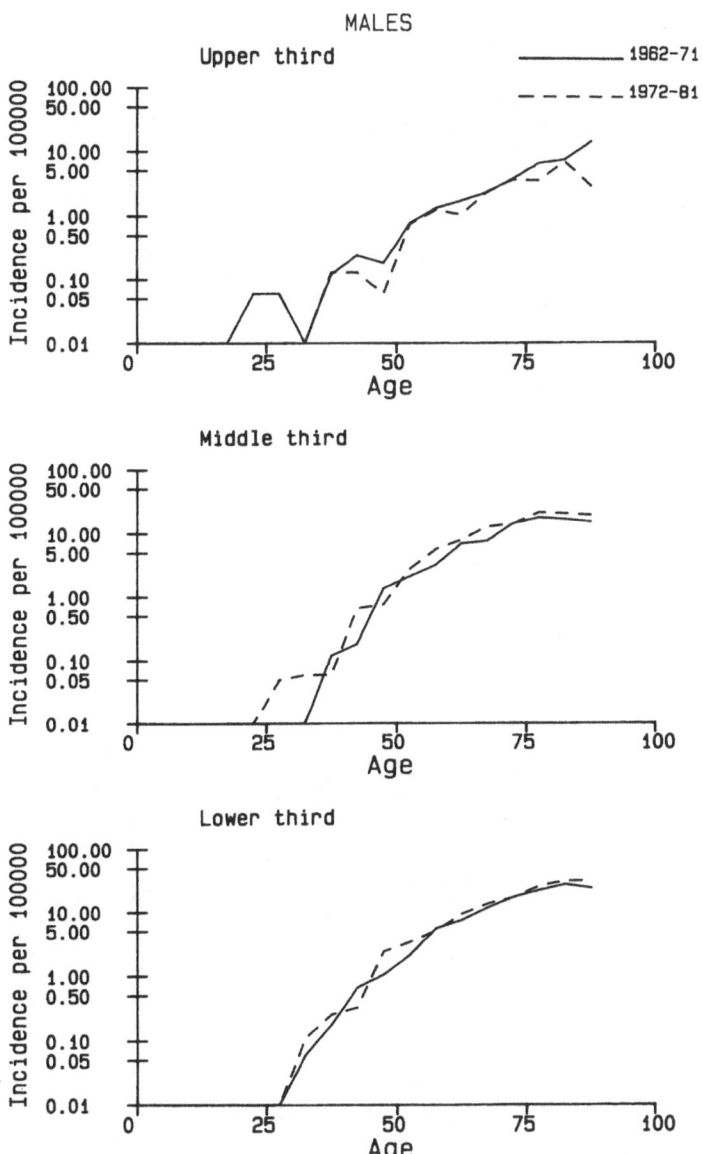

Figure 2.12.1 Incidence Rates by Age, Site, Sex and Decade.

Table 2.12.2 Incidence Rates by Age, Site and Sex. Decade 1972-81.

Age group	Upper third		Middle third		Lower third		Site unspecified	
	Male	Female	Male	Female	Male	Female	Male	Female
0 – 19	–	–	–	–	–	–	–	–
20 – 24	–	–	–	0.06	–	–	–	–
25 – 29	–	–	0.05	–	–	–	–	–
30 – 34	–	–	0.06	0.24	0.11	0.07	–	–
35 – 39	0.13	0.13	0.06	0.27	0.26	0.41	0.06	–
40 – 44	0.13	0.14	0.66	0.55	0.33	0.79	0.13	0.14
45 – 49	0.06	0.13	0.76	1.05	2.41	2.41	–	–
50 – 54	0.74	0.43	2.78	3.09	3.33	3.05	0.37	0.31
55 – 59	1.23	1.19	5.68	4.05	5.13	4.14	0.82	0.33
60 – 64	1.04	0.62	7.97	6.08	9.31	5.03	0.97	1.04
65 – 69	2.35	2.06	12.66	6.86	13.56	8.16	2.44	1.22
70 – 74	3.53	1.48	14.10	8.44	17.10	13.65	3.79	2.13
75 – 79	3.41	1.82	21.41	11.44	26.28	16.23	7.54	3.64
80 – 84	6.70	1.97	20.62	12.94	31.44	17.67	8.25	5.04
85 – 89	2.78	3.26	19.44	13.49	31.94	12.68	15.28	12.56
90 – 94	–	2.82	15.79	15.49	31.58	5.88	31.58	15.49
95+	–	5.88	–	11.77	50.00	–	25.00	17.65
All ages	0.51	0.44	2.55	2.30	3.07	2.08	0.61	0.60

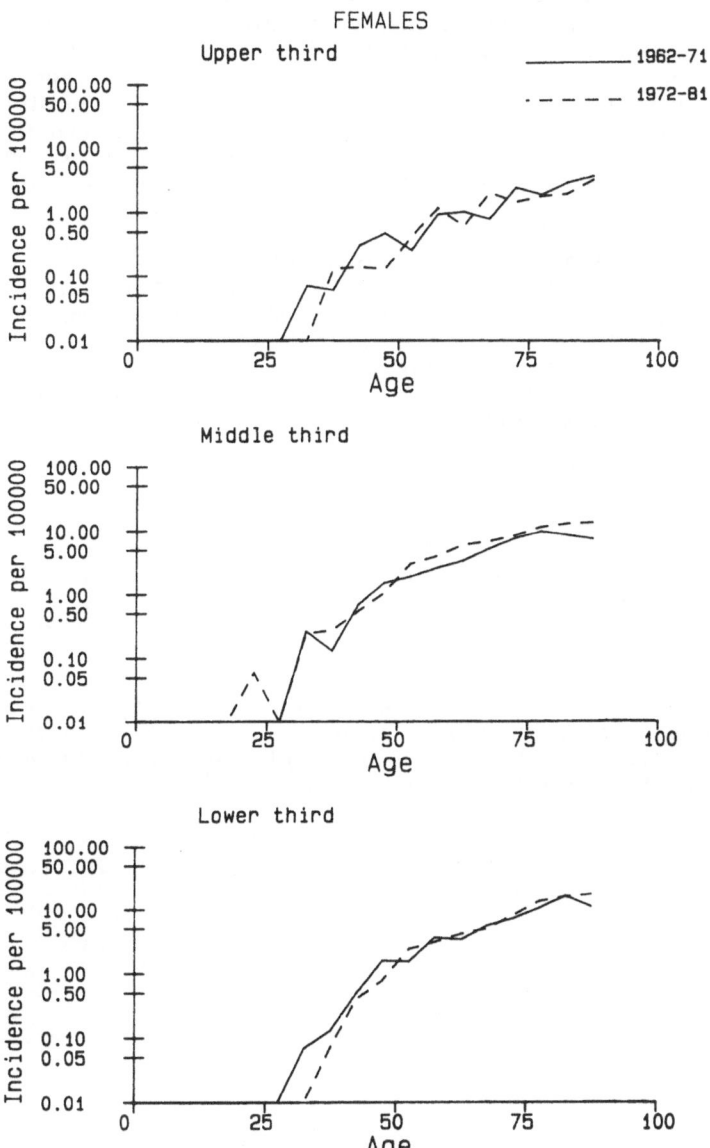

Figure 2.12.2   Incidence Rates by Age, Site, Sex and Decade.

Figure 2.13 - Incidence Rates in Cohorts by Central Year of Birth

It is often helpful, when age incidence rates are available over an extended period of time, to examine the trends in relation to age for groups of people born at different times.   For convenience, such groups are called cohorts in epidemiological parlance and they are usually described by their 'central year of birth'.   For instance, a group of people with a certain incidence rate in 1964 at age 50-54, will have a different (and higher) rate 5 years later (in 1969) when they are at age 55-59; 10 years later still (in 1979) at age 65-69, they will have an even higher rate, but they will still constitute the same basic cohort, even though there will have been losses through death.   This cohort would be described as the 1912 cohort, because it includes those born in the years 1910-1914, the central year being 1912.

For males, the four oldest cohorts overlie one another, except possibly for the oldest of all, born in 1875.   Subsequent cohorts show a steadily increasing risk.   For females, again except for the oldest of all (1875), which resembles that for males, each success-ively later-born cohort shows higher rates than the previous one. The youngest two are not yet sufficient in numbers of cases to be able to discern their pattern.

Technical Note

In Figures 2.13.1 and 2.13.2 the points each represent a 10-year age group observed in a quinquennium.   For example, the point denoted by the open square represents the age group 20-29 in the quinquennium 1957-1961.   The full range of birth years is thus 1928-1941, the central year of which has been taken to be 1935. Successive points are plotted at yearly intervals of age, so that they include overlapping 10-year age groups, the next to 20-29 being 25-34, etc.   This procedure has been adopted because otherwise the numbers would be too small and unstable.

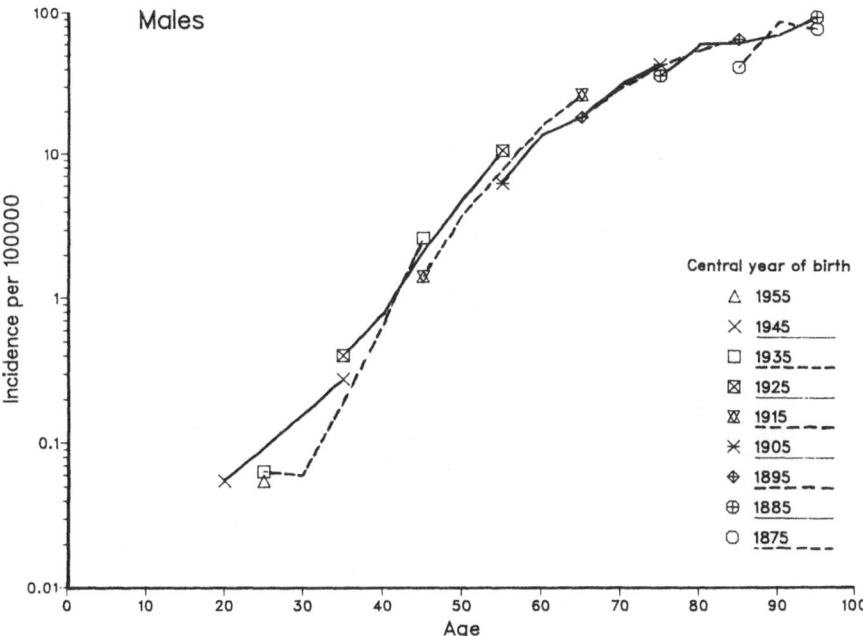

Figure 2.13.1   Incidence Rates in Cohorts (males).

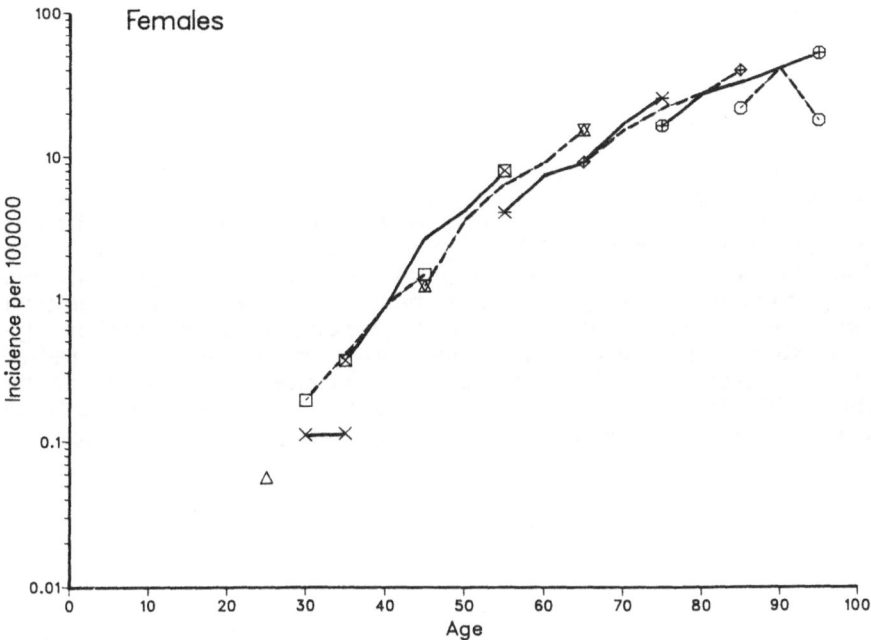

Figure 2.13.2   Incidence Rates in Cohorts (females).

3

Histology

Data relating to the whole population of 6398 patients is given in Table 3.1. From Table 3.3 onwards the 25 'atypical' tumours are excluded, until they are considered as a separate group in Chapter 7. The remaining cases are then analysed with respect to numbers and incidence rates for the different histological categories, by site and sex, for individual years, for quinquennia and for the age of the patient.

3.1 SUMMARY OF FINDINGS

The numbers of cases of the three major histological types are sufficiently large to permit useful analysis and comparison in several ways, as this chapter demonstrates. It is interesting, for instance, that the proportion of males with adenocarcinoma is about twice that of females, and that this ratio is similar for both the middle and lower thirds. Moreover, the proportion of adenocarcinomas has increased steadily in both sexes over the period of study, and this is despite the very careful scrutiny and exclusion of tumours of the cardia. The fact that the increases with time are highly significant in both sexes when expressed as proportions (Table 3.5), but are only so for males when comparing age-standardised rates (Table 3.7), is explained simply by the fact that the World Standard Population has only a relatively small proportion in the higher age groups, where the increase has been most noticeable; the smaller numbers of cases of adenocarcinoma in females than males, taken together with the very late age distribution of female cases (see Table 3.9), accounts for the difference in statistical significance.

Table 3.1

The proportion of cases with unspecified or no histology probably
reflects the late stage of the disease at presentation in many patients
and can be correlated with the fact that a large number did not
receive any anti-tumour treatment (see Chapter 5). The proportion
of cases with no histology has, however, diminished over time, from
34% in the first quinquennium to 27% in the fifth. All cases where
the diagnosis of malignancy might have been incorrect were individually reviewed, as indicated in Chapter 1.

Table 3.1 Histological Categories.

	No	%	%
Carcinoma	4321	97.3	
Malignant, type not specified	61	1.4	
Suggestive of malignancy	41	0.9	
Melanoma	1	0.02	
Sarcoma	17	0.4	
Total with histology	4441	100.0	69.4
No histology	1957		30.6
All cases	6398		100.0

Table 3.2

This data relates to the 4339 cases in which the histological type was specified, and indicates that primary tumours other than squamous, anaplastic and adenocarcinomas are extremely rare - averaging only one case per annum for the whole region.   In view of this finding these 25 'atypical' tumours are excluded from all subsequent analyses and are considered as a separate group in Chapter 7.   It should be emphasised that the proportion of adenocarcinomas (11.9%) represents a 'true' incidence of this tumour in the oesophagus, as tumours of the cardia have been specifically excluded from this survey (see Chapter 1).

Table 3.2 Numbers and Distribution (%) - Histological Type Specified.

	Histology from primary		Histology from secondary		All sources	
	No.	%	No.	%	No.	%
Squamous cell carcinoma	3348	79.0	59	59.0	3407	78.5
Adenocarcinoma	500	11.8	18	18.0	518	11.9
Adeno-squamous carcinoma	9	0.2	0	0.0	9	0.2
Anaplastic carcinoma	358	8.4	22	22.0	380	8.8
Other Tumours	24	0.6	1	1.0	25	0.6
Transitional cell carcinoma	3		0		3	
Basal cell carcinoma	1		0		1	
Carcinoid	1		0		1	
Pseudosarcoma	3		0		3	
Melanoma	1		0		1	
Sarcoma	15		1		16	
		100.0		100.0		100.0

Table 3.3.1.

This data relates to the 6373 cases remaining after exclusion of the 25 'atypical' tumours which are considered separately in Chapter 7.

Table 3.3.1. Numbers by Histology, Site and Sex.

	Upper third		Middle third		Lower third		Site unspecified	
	M	F	M	F	M	F	M	F
Squamous cell carcinoma	207	190	769	740	684	601	119	97
Adenocarcinoma	5	7	102	53	241	84	15	11
Adeno-squamous carcinoma	3	0	1	1	1	2	1	0
Anaplastic carcinoma	13	7	78	89	112	60	11	10
Malignant, type not specified	0	3	9	7	23	9	6	4
Suggestive of malignancy	3	3	9	4	15	4	2	1
Total with histology	231	210	968	894	1076	760	154	123
No histology	84	60	291	215	480	348	259	220

Table 3.3.2

The proportion of males with adenocarcinoma is approximately twice that of females, for both middle and lower thirds; in each case these differences are very highly significant.

Table 3.3.2 Distribution (%) by Histology, Site and Sex.

	Upper third		Middle third		Lower third		Site unspecified	
	M	F	M	F	M	F	M	F
Squamous cell carcinoma	89.6	90.6	79.5	82.8	63.6	79.1	77.3	78.9
Adenocarcinoma	2.2	3.3	10.5***	5.9***	22.4+++	11.0+++	9.7	8.9
Adeno-squamous carcinoma	1.3	0.0	0.1	0.1	0.1	0.3	0.6	0.0
Anaplastic carcinoma	5.6	3.3	8.1	10.0	10.4	7.9	7.2	8.1
Malignant, type not specified	0.0	1.4	0.9	0.8	2.1	1.2	3.9	3.3
Suggestive of malignancy	1.3	1.4	0.9	0.4	1.4	0.5	1.3	0.8
Total with histology	100.0	100.0	100.0	100.0	100.0	100.0	100.0	100.0
No histology as % of all cases	26.7	22.2	23.1	19.4	30.8	31.4	62.7	64.1

Table 3.4

This data and subsequent data in this chapter relates to the 4305 cases with tumours of the three major histological types, excluding the nine mixed adeno-squamous tumours.

Table 3.4   Numbers per Annum by Histology and Sex.

Year	Squamous cell Male	Squamous cell Female	Adenocarcinoma Male	Adenocarcinoma Female	Anaplastic Male	Anaplastic Female
1957	49	35	4	3	4	1
1958	53	37	5	3	8	2
1959	55	52	7	0	5	4
1960	49	41	3	1	10	3
1961	49	47	3	5	8	6
1957–61	255	212	22	12	35	16
1962	68	54	1	4	5	6
1963	76	60	5	3	1	5
1964	68	56	7	1	4	2
1965	60	61	11	5	5	7
1966	75	54	7	4	9	6
1962–66	347	285	31	17	24	26
1967	58	54	8	6	9	3
1968	65	62	10	7	10	7
1969	62	80	10	3	7	4
1970	85	69	5	3	6	6
1971	69	66	8	4	11	6
1967–71	339	331	41	23	43	26
1972	82	84	15	1	12	4
1973	65	73	18	5	17	10
1974	87	66	15	12	6	5
1975	79	68	19	11	15	14
1976	101	89	28	13	9	9
1972–76	414	380	95	42	59	42
1977	80	84	38	13	10	15
1978	83	82	34	15	16	15
1979	90	79	21	9	8	8
1980	82	91	37	11	10	11
1981	89	84	44	13	9	7
1977–81	424	420	174	61	53	56
1957–81	1779	1628	363	155	214	166

Table 3.5

The increase in the proportion of adenocarcinomas from the second to the fifth quinquennium is, for each sex, statistically significant; the second quinquennium has been taken as the baseline rather than the first as there was known to be under-registration in the first quinquennium, although we have no reason to believe that this was biased towards or against any specific histology. It is possible that this may reflect a rise in the incidence of columnar-lined oeso-phagus, though this cannot be determined from our data. There is, of course, a corresponding fall in the proportion of squamous tumours. The numbers of cases of anaplastic carcinoma are too small to attain statistical significance.

Table 3.5 Distribution (%) by Quinquennium, Histology and Sex.

Years	Squamous cell carcinoma		Adenocarcinoma		Anaplastic carcinoma		Total of these histologies	
	Male %	Female %	Male %	Female %	Male %	Female %	Male %	Female %
1957-61	81.7	88.3	7.1	5.0	11.2	6.7	100.0	100.0
1962-66	86.3	86.9	7.7***	5.2**	6.0	7.9	100.0	100.0
1967-71	80.1	87.1	9.7	6.1	10.2	6.8	100.0	100.0
1972-76	72.9	81.8	16.7	9.1	10.4	9.1	100.0	100.0
1977-81	65.1	78.2	26.7***	11.4**	8.2	10.4	100.0	100.0
1957-81	75.5	83.5	15.4	8.0	9.1	8.5	100.0	100.0

Table 3.6

These rates show an increase in the incidence of squamous carcinoma for both sexes in the middle third and for women in the lower third. For all sites taken together there has been an increase in both sexes but the differences (between the second and fifth quinquennia) are not significant.

Table 3.6 Age Standardised Incidence Rates by Quinquennium, Site and Sex.

SQUAMOUS CELL CARCINOMA

Quinquennium	Upper third M	Upper third F	Middle third M	Middle third F	Lower third M	Lower third F	Site unspec M	Site unspec F	All sites M	All sites F
1957 – 61	0.137	0.195	0.651	0.445	0.727	0.434	0.314	0.102	1.829	1.176
1962 – 66	0.366	0.222	0.782	0.643	1.002	0.585	0.137	0.060	2.287	1.509
1967 – 71	0.272	0.167	0.948	0.703	0.771	0.689	0.092	0.057	2.083	1.616
1972 – 76	0.229	0.198	1.164	0.878	0.842	0.543	0.096	0.143	2.331	1.762
1977 – 81	0.269	0.183	1.095	0.967	0.844	0.677	0.111	0.069	2.319	1.896

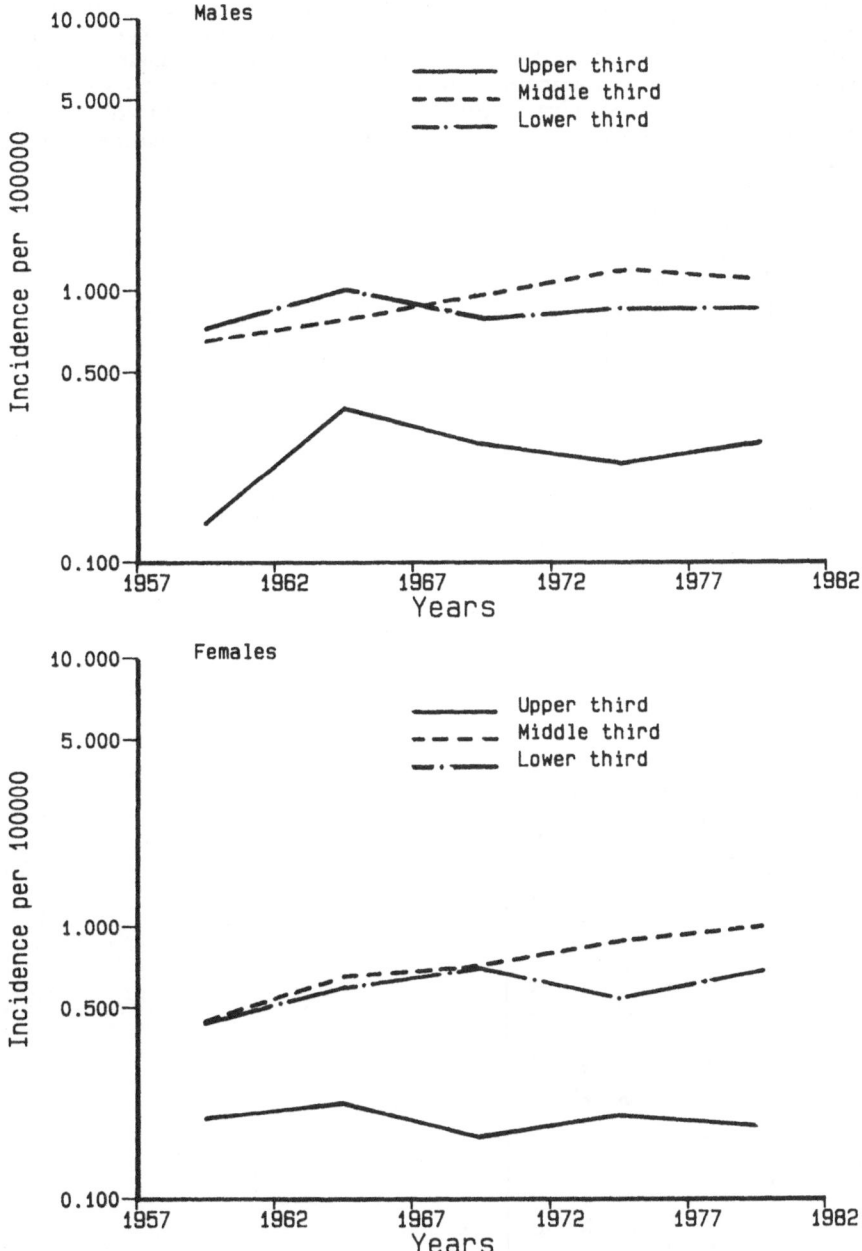

Figure 3.6   Squamous - Incidence by Quinquennium, Site and Sex.

Clinical Cancer Monographs: Oesophagus

Table 3.7

For adenocarcinomas there is a highly significant increase in males in the lower third; there is also an increased rate in females but this is not significant. These findings are reflected in the increased rates for all sites in both sexes but here the difference in males is very highly significant. Adenocarcinomas of the upper third are extremely uncommon and show no significant change. Clearly the increase in the middle third cannot be due to miscoding of tumours of the cardia.

Table 3.7 Age Standardised Incidence Rates by Quinquennium, Site and Sex.

Quinquennium	ADENOCARCINOMA									
	Upper third		Middle third		Lower third		Site unspec.		All sites	
	M	F	M	F	M	F	M	F	M	F
1957 – 61	0.000	0.006	0.050	0.019	0.097	0.026	0.008	0.010	0.155	0.060
1962 – 66	0.011	0.003	0.033	0.030	0.153**	0.049	0.007	0.000	0.204***	0.082
1967 – 71	0.005	0.003	0.049	0.038	0.204	0.055	0.000	0.000	0.258	0.095
1972 – 76	0.000	0.010	0.176	0.052	0.353	0.093	0.018	0.016	0.546	0.171
1977 – 81	0.011	0.005	0.287	0.096.	0.648**	0.126	0.047	0.017	0.994***	0.244

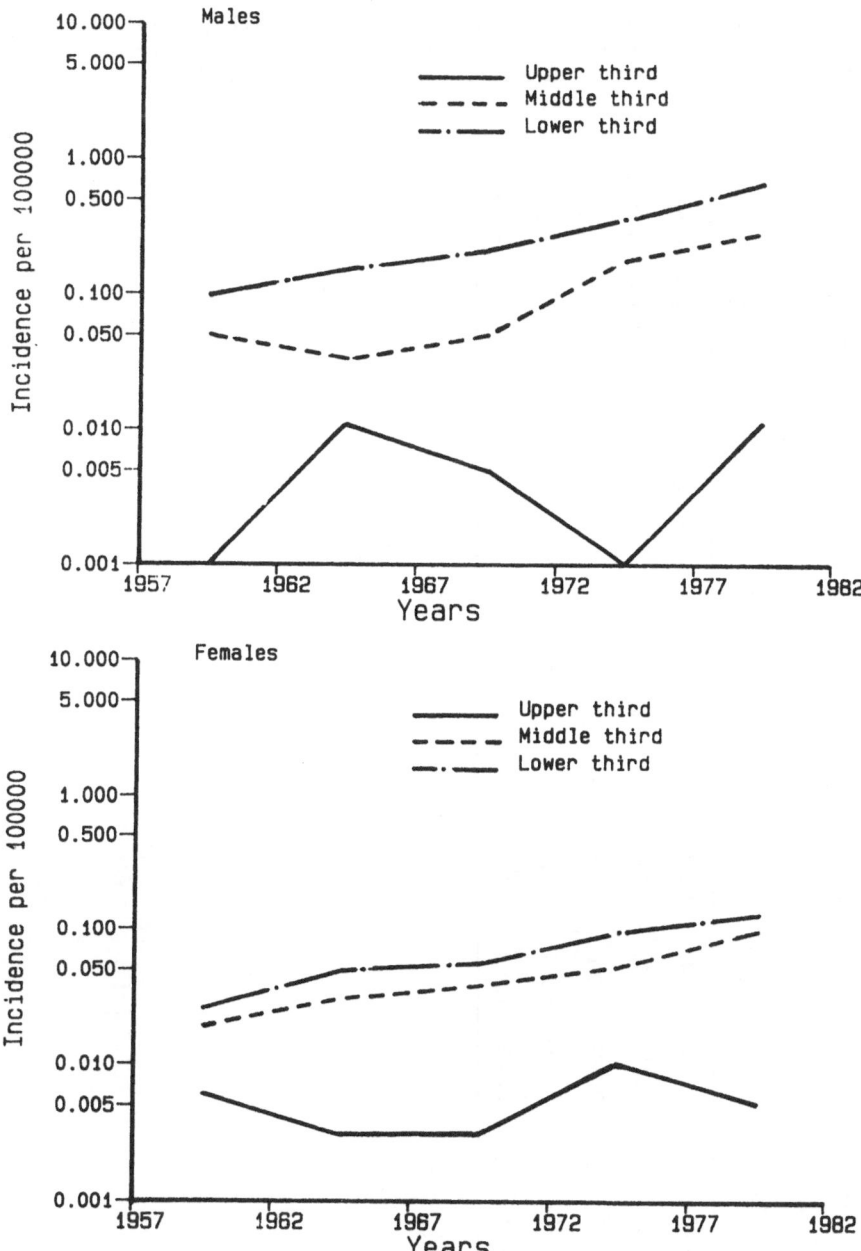

Figure 3.7   Adenocarcinoma - Incidence by Quinquennium, Site and Sex.

Table 3.8

For anaplastic carcinomas there has been an increase in the middle third for females but the lower third shows little change in either sex. For all sites there has been an increase for both sexes but the numbers are too small to attain statistical significance.

Table 3.8   Age Standardised Incidence Rates by Quinquennium, Site and Sex.

ANAPLASTIC CARCINOMA

Quinquennium	Upper third M	F	Middle third M	F	Lower third M	F	Site unspec. M	F	All sites M	F
1957 – 61	0.016	0.000	0.086	0.043	0.117	0.029	0.029	0.011	0.248	0.083
1962 – 66	0.013	0.010	0.063	0.062	0.084	0.055	0.000	0.000	0.159	0.128
1967 – 71	0.023	0.000	0.088	0.057	0.146	0.051	0.000	0.012	0.257	0.120
1972 – 76	0.015	0.009	0.116	0.149	0.150	0.063	0.016	0.008	0.298	0.229
1977 – 81	0.015	0.009	0.116	0.149	0.150	0.063	0.016	0.008	0.298	0.229

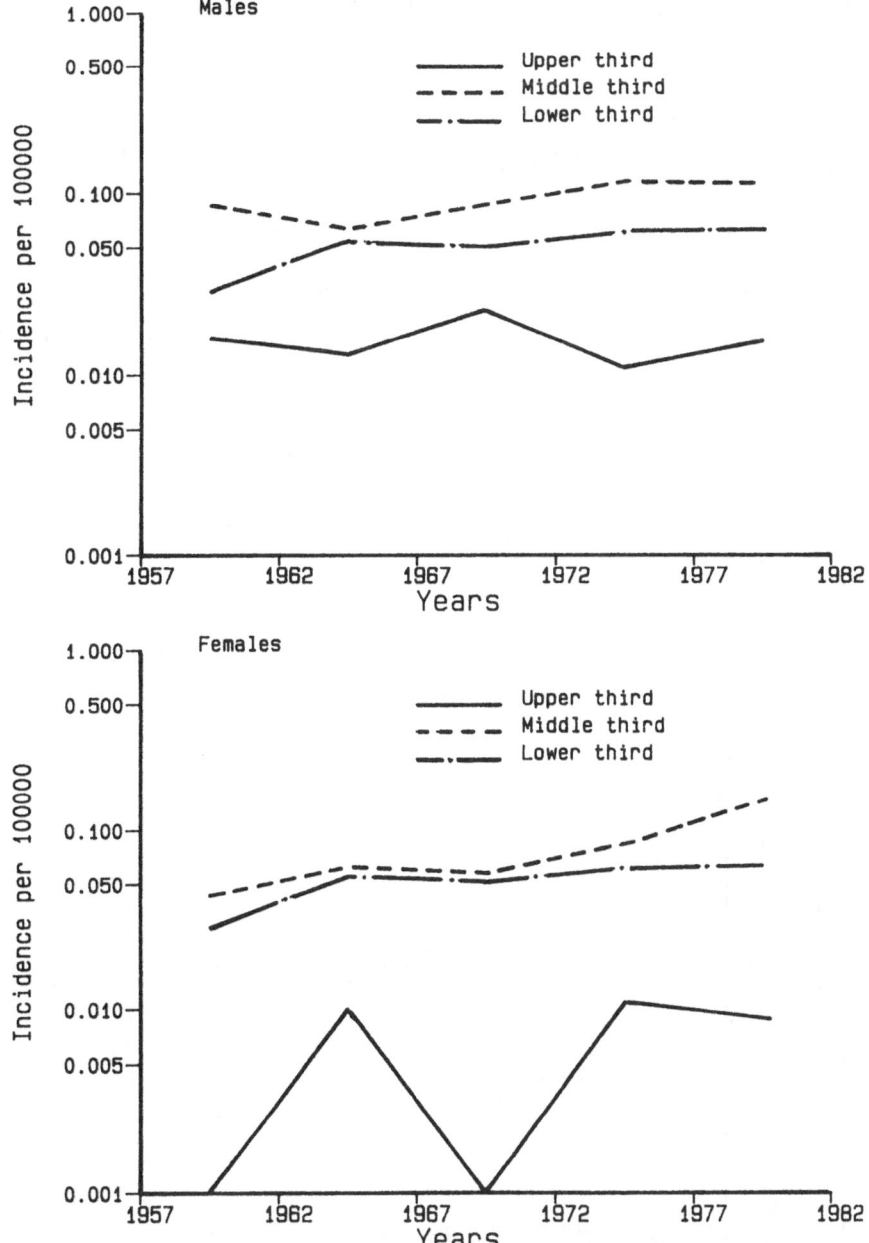

Figure 3.8   Anaplastic - Incidence by Quinquennium, Site and Sex.

Table 3.9

These numbers are given for completeness in order to allow the reader to calculate different age groups as desired.

Table 3.9 Numbers by Age, Histology and Sex.

Age group	Squamous cell carcinoma Male No.	Squamous cell carcinoma Female No.	Adenocarcinoma Male No.	Adenocarcinoma Female No.	Anaplastic carcinoma Male No.	Anaplastic carcinoma Female No.	Total of these histologies Male No.	Total of these histologies Female No.
0 – 19	0	0	0	0	0	0	0	0
20 – 24	1	0	0	1	0	0	1	1
25 – 29	2	0	1	0	0	0	3	0
30 – 34	4	11	1	0	0	1	5	12
35 – 39	16	15	1	1	0	0	17	16
40 – 44	26	39	6	3	2	2	34	44
45 – 49	63	88	25	1	12	5	100	94
50 – 54	136	160	41	9	19	8	196	177
55 – 59	242	203	45	13	26	18	313	234
60 – 64	302	229	65	17	31	14	398	260
65 – 69	359	253	75	22	45	37	479	312
70 – 74	310	262	44	29	35	30	389	321
75 – 79	198	207	40	34	27	26	265	267
80 – 84	90	97	13	14	11	14	114	125
85 – 89	24	54	2	6	5	7	31	67
90 – 94	5	10	3	5	1	3	9	18
95+	1	0	0	0	0	1	1	1
Unknown	0	0	1	0	0	0	1	0
All ages	1779	1628	363	155	214	166	2356	1949

Table 3.10

The distribution of the major histological types of tumour shows no consistent change with age.

Table 3.10 Distribution (%) by Age, Sex and Histology.

Age group	Males				Females			
	Squamous	Adenocarc.	Anaplastic		Squamous	Adenocarc.	Anaplastic	
20 - 29	75.0	25.0	0.0	100.0	0.0	100.0	0.0	100.0
30 - 39	90.9	9.1	0.0	100.0	92.8	3.6	3.6	100.0
40 - 49	66.4	23.1	10.5	100.0	92.0	2.9	5.1	100.0
50 - 59	74.3	16.9	8.8	100.0	88.3	5.4	6.3	100.0
60 - 69	75.4	15.9	8.7	100.0	84.3	6.8	8.9	100.0
70 - 79	77.7	12.8	9.5	100.0	79.8	10.7	9.5	100.0
80 - 89	78.6	10.4	11.0	100.0	78.7	10.4	10.9	100.0
90+	60.0	30.0	10.0	100.0	52.6	26.3	21.1	100.0
All ages	75.5	15.4	9.1	100.0	83.5	8.0	8.5	100.0

Table 3.11 Mean Age (years) by Quinquennium, Histology and Sex.

Year	Squamous		Adenocarcinoma		Anaplastic	
	Mean age		Mean age		Mean age	
	Male	Female	Male	Female	Male	Female
1957–61	65.2	64.3	64.8	69.6	64.6	65.9
1962–66	65.2	64.7	63.6	66.9	67.1	66.2
1967–71	65.0	65.2	63.6	71.4	66.1	68.5
1972–76	66.1	65.8	63.3	70.4	65.6	72.0
1977–81	66.9	67.2	64.8	70.7	68.0	70.3
1957–81	65.8	65.7	64.1	70.2	66.3	69.4

4

Overall Survival

In order to allow 5-year survival rates to be calculated, data in this chapter relates to the 4680 tumours which were registered from 1957 to 1976 (excluding the 22 atypical tumours that occurred during this period). Survival rates have been calculated according to the method described in Chapter 1 (and in Appendix 2) and analysed with respect to histology, age, site, sex and quinquennium. The five cases of mixed adeno-squamous tumour are excluded from analyses which are histology specific.

In some cases, both arithmetic and logarithmic scales have been used to illustrate the results. The general reasons for using logarithmic scales for the vertical measurement are discussed in Chapter 1. In this chapter logarithmic scales have been used to enable the differences in survival to be seen more clearly.

4.1 SUMMARY OF FINDINGS

Survival is very poor (3% overall at 5 years), but females survive, in general, rather better than males. There is no appreciable difference between the three subsites in terms of survival. Histologically, squamous carcinomas survive better than adenocarcinomas, and each better than the anaplastic tumours. Survival rates tend to fall off sharply with increasing age. It is disappointing to have to record that there has been no noticeable improvement in survival over the 20-year period analysed here, despite the changes in treatment that have taken place. Chapter 6 will show that a significant improvement in the survival rate occurs only among upper third tumours treated by radiotherapy.

Table 4.1

This data emphasises that carcinoma of the oesophagus is a very lethal tumour. Less than 15% of patients were alive at 1 year (whether crude or age-adjusted rates are used) and this is in spite of the fact that approximately 28% had radical treatment and 41% had some form of therapy directed at the primary tumour (see Chapter 5). After the first year, mortality rates decline progressively, with approximately 50% of those remaining, dying in the second year and just over a quarter dying in the third year. Allowance for the increasing general mortality with age, shown by the age-adjusted survival rate, increases the crude survival rate by a proportion which varies from about 5% to 19%, but makes little visible difference to the survival curve (Figure 4.1).

Table 4.1   Annual Crude and Age Adjusted Survival Rates for 4680 Patients.

| | Survival in years | | | | |
	1	2	3	4	5
Number alive	635	297	210	162	148
Crude survival rate(%)	13.6	6.3	4.5	3.5	3.2
Age adjusted survival rate (%)	14.3	6.9	5.1	4.0	3.8

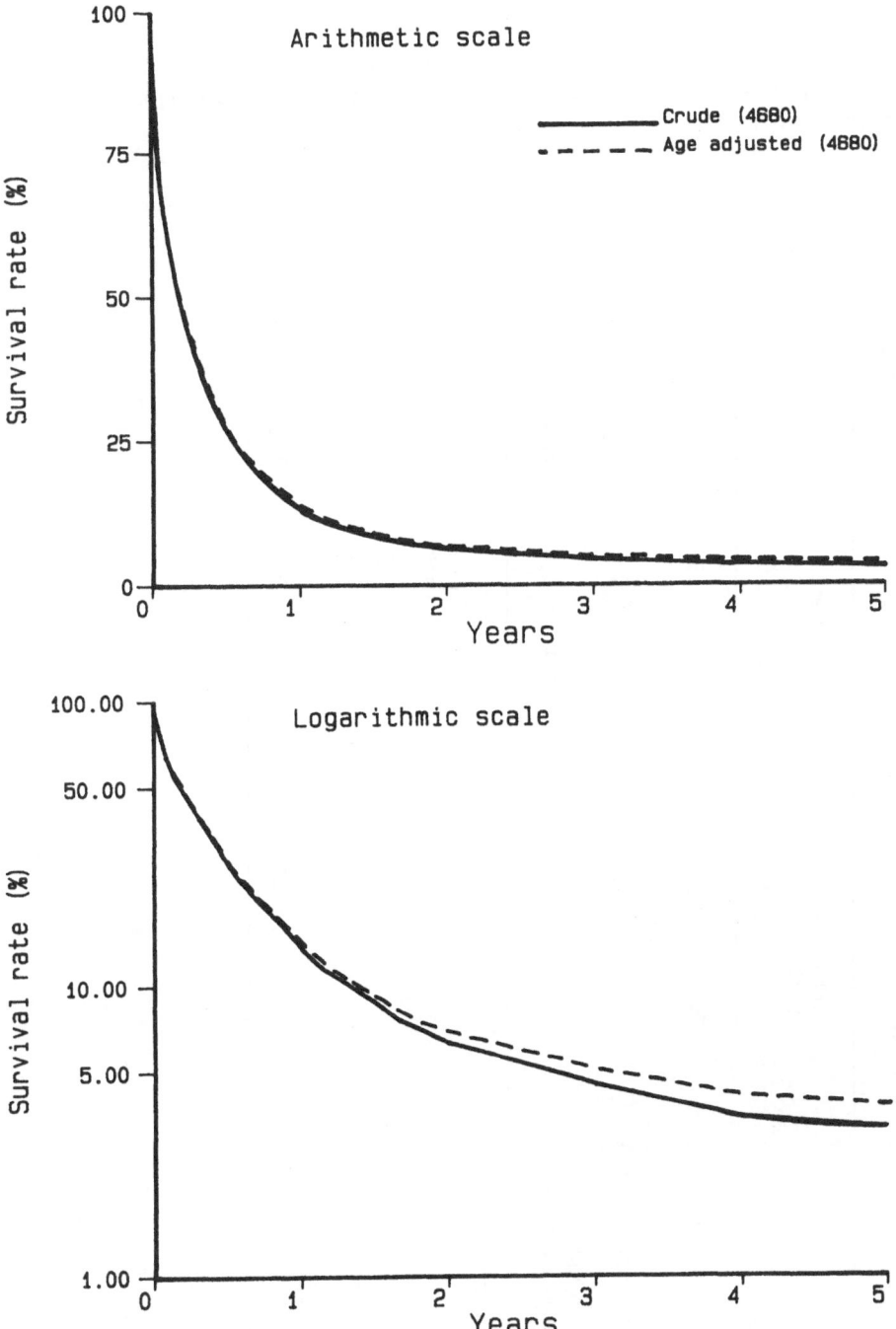

Figure 4.1   Annual Rates, Crude and Age Adjusted.

Table 4.2

The poorer survival rate of males is clearly shown here and is very highly significant at both 1 and 5 years; the divergence also increases with time.

Table 4.2 Annual Crude and Age Adjusted Survival Rates by Sex for 4680 Patients.

	Total number	Survival in years				
		1	2	3	4	5
MALES						
Number alive	2620	297	121	77	54	46
Crude survival rate (%)		11.3	4.6	2.9	2.1	1.8
Age adjusted survival rate(%)		12.0***	5.1	3.4	2.5	2.2+++
FEMALES						
Number alive	2060	338	176	133	108	102
Crude survival rate (%)		16.4	8.5	6.5	5.2	5.0
Age adjusted survival rate (%)		17.2***	9.2	7.1	5.9	5.7+++

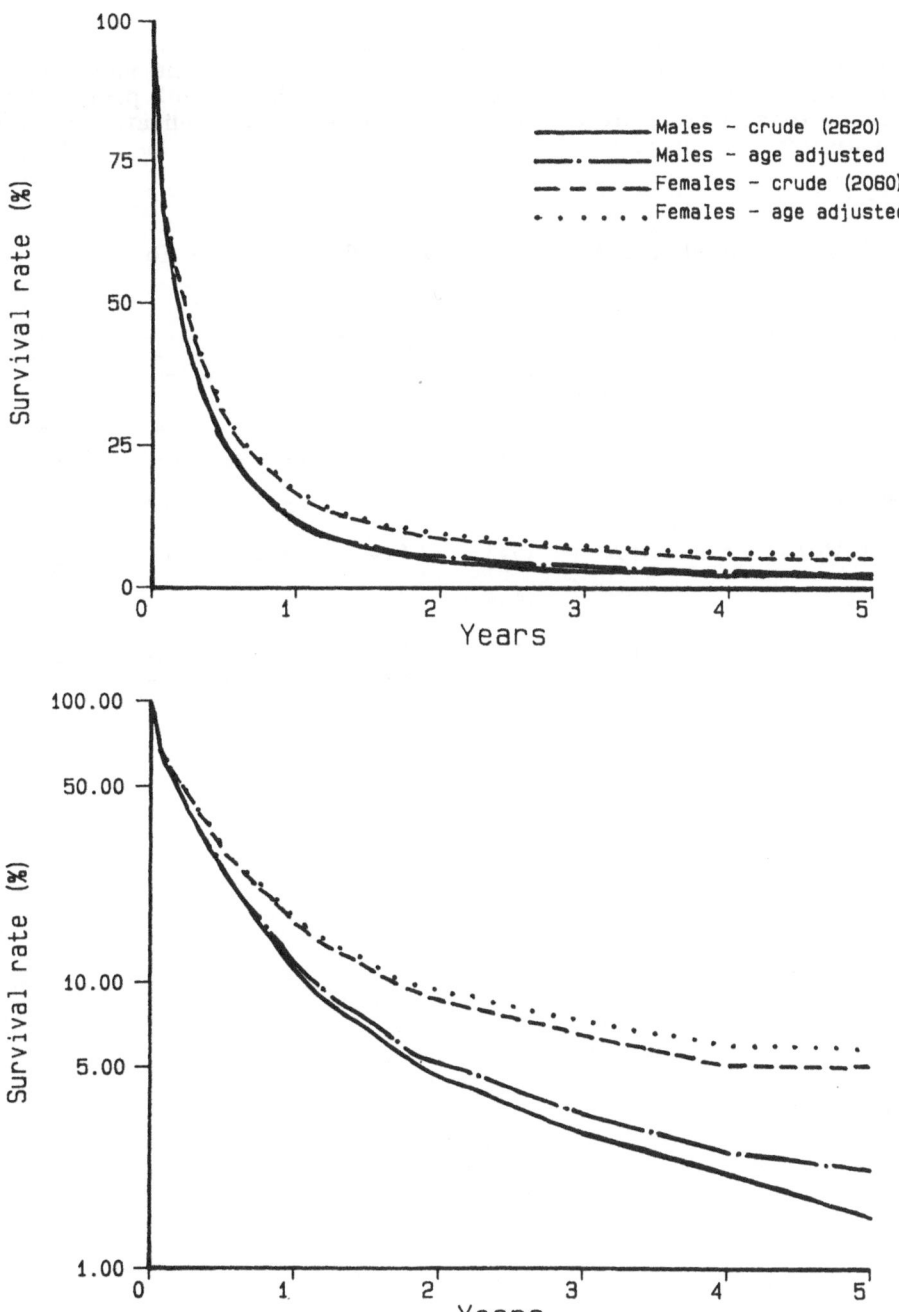

Figure 4.2   Annual Rates, Crude and Age Adjusted by Sex.

Table 4.3

Contrary to some statements in the literature there is no significant difference between the sites in their survival rates. The survival of those where the site was not specified is much poorer, presumably because these were more advanced cases where the localisation of the tumour was less precise.

Table 4.3   Annual Age Adjusted Survival Rates by Site for 4680
             Patients.

Site	Total number	% survival in years				
		1	2	3	4	5
Upper third	459	16.1	6.7	5.2	4.8	4.5
Middle third	1692	15.3	6.9	5.0	4.0	3.6
Lower third	1927	15.8	8.3	6.2	4.9	4.8
Site unspecified	602	5.2	2.8	1.4	0.4	0.4

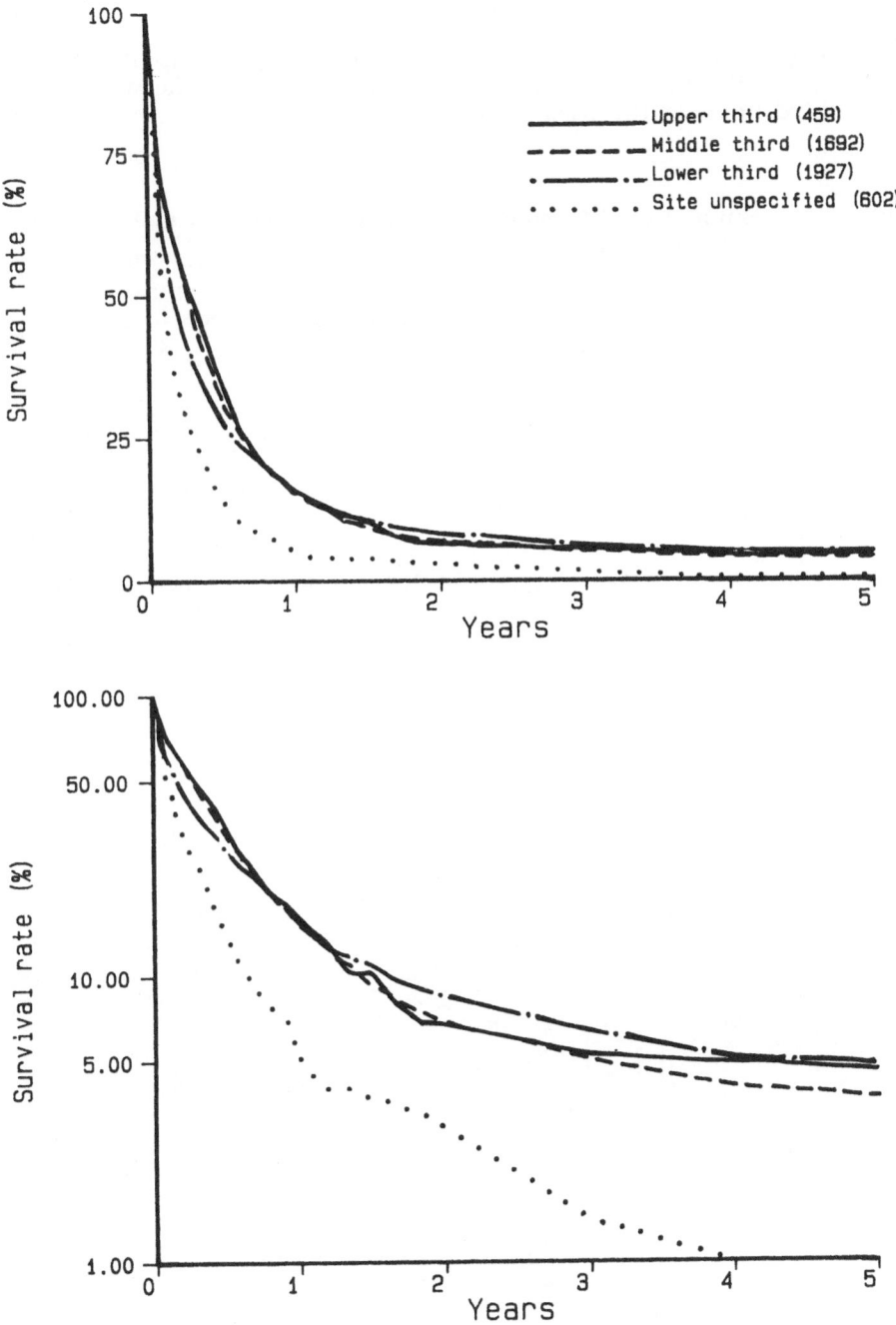

Figure 4.3   Annual Rates by Site.

Table 4.4

When the site-specific survival rates are subdivided by sex, the poorer 5-year survival rate in males is very highly significant for both the middle and lower thirds, but only just significant for the upper third, due to the smaller numbers of cases.

Table 4.4   Annual Age Adjusted Survival Rates by Site and by Sex for 4680 Patients.

Site		Total number	% survival in years				
			1	2	3	4	5
Upper third	M	240	12.4	4.2	2.4	2.5	2.0*
	F	219	20.0	9.4	8.1	7.4	7.1*
Middle third	M	920	12.8	4.9	3.6	2.3	1.9***
	F	772	18.3	9.1	6.6	5.9	5.6***
Lower third	M	1124	13.3	6.3	4.1	3.2	3.0+++
	F	803	19.3	11.1	9.1	7.4	7.3+++
Site unspecified	M	336	5.5	2.4	1.1	0.4	0.4
	F	266	4.9	3.3	1.7	0.4	0.5

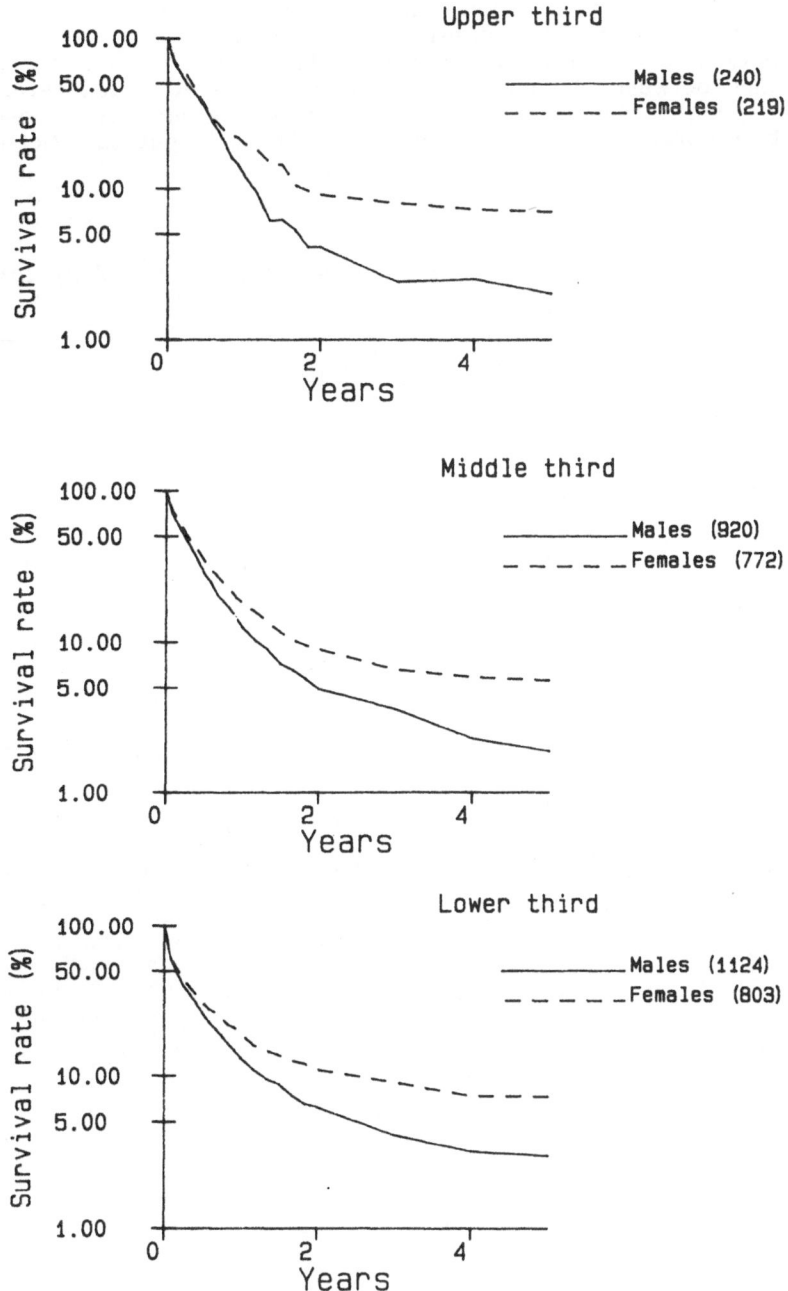

Figure 4.4   Annual Rates by Site and Sex.

Table 4.5

Squamous cell carcinoma shows the best survival rates, which at 5 years are very highly significantly different from both adeno-carcinomas and anaplastic carcinomas. There is in fact a significant difference between the survival rates at 1 year for adenocarcinomas and anaplastic carcinomas, but this diminishes and at 5 years is actually reversed, though that difference is no longer significant.

Table 4.5   Annual Age Adjusted Survival Rates by Histology for 4680 Patients.

Histology	Total number	% survival in years				
		1	2	3	4	5
Squamous cell carcinoma	2563	20.4	10.4	7.9	6.6	6.3*** +++
Adenocarcinoma	283	17.0	6.8	4.7	1.6	0.8***
Adeno-squamous carcinoma	5	20.9	0.0	0.0	0.0	0.0
Anaplastic carcinoma	271	8.9	3.2	2.1	1.8	1.4+++
Malignant, type not specified	27	15.8	8.1	4.2	4.3	4.5
Suggestive of carcinoma	32	6.7	3.6	3.6	3.7	3.7
No histology	1499	4.0	1.5	0.6	0.3	0.3

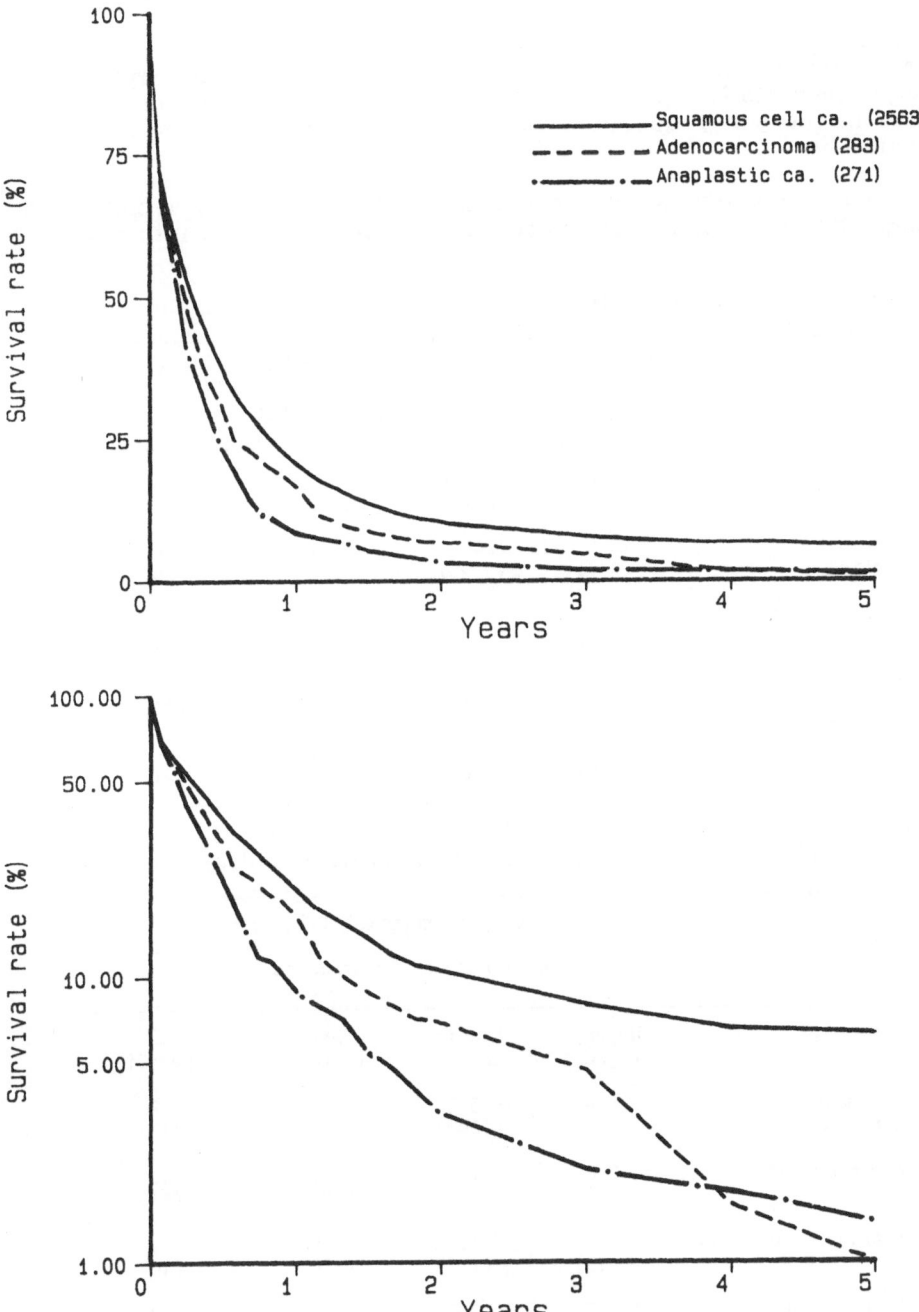

Figure 4.5   Annual Rates by Histology.

Table 4.6

The differences in survival rates here, whether at 1 year or 5 years, reflect those already discussed for site or histology separately; their statistical significance depends rather on the numbers of cases in the subgroups, and for that reason has not been evaluated separately.

The adeno-squamous carcinomas, 'type not specified' and 'suggestive of malignancy' categories are not subdivided into sites.

Table 4.6.1 Age Adjusted Survival Rates by Histology and Site.

| | One year survival (%) | | | |
| | Total numbers in brackets | | | |
Histology	Upper third	Middle third	Lower third	Site unspecified
Squamous cell carcinoma	18.6 (307)	20.1 (1098)	23.3 (983)	9.6 (175)
Adenocarcinoma	11.9 (9)	15.3 (82)	17.3 (181)	28.4 (11)
Anaplastic carcinoma	7.0 (15)	9.5 (110)	8.9 (130)	6.5 (16)
No histology	9.2 (118)	3.3 (384)	4.5 (606)	2.5 (391)

Table 4.6.2 Age Adjusted Survival Rates by Histology and Site.

| | Five year survival (%) | | | |
| | Total numbers in brackets | | | |
Histology	Upper third	Middle third	Lower third	Site unspecified
Squamous cell carcinoma	5.4 (307)	5.3 (1098)	8.5 (983)	1.3 (175)
Adenocarcinoma	0.0 (9)	1.4 (82)	0.7 (181)	0.0 (11)
Anaplastic carcinoma	0.0 (15)	1.1 (110)	1.9 (130)	0.0 (16)
No histology	2.5 (118)	0.0 (384)	0.3 (606)	0.0 (391)

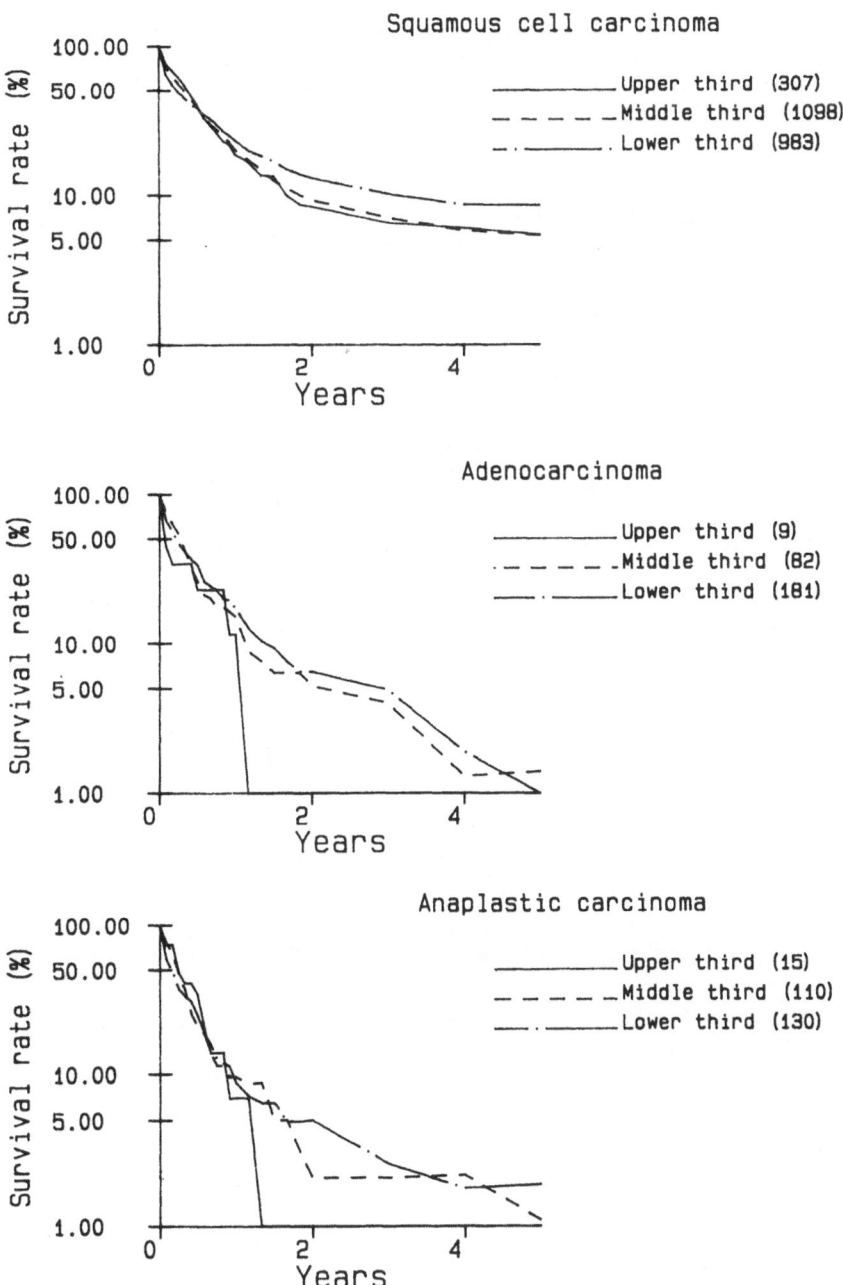

Figure 4.6   Annual Rates by Histology and Site.

Table 4.7

As in Table 4.4, the differences between the sexes in survival rates
for squamous cell carcinoma at 5 years are very highly significant
statistically for middle and lower thirds, but only just significant for
the upper third. The differences between sites within the same sex
are not significant.

Table 4.7   Squamous Cell Carcinoma.
            Age Adjusted Survival Rates (%) by Site and Sex.

	Males			Females		
	Total number	One year	Five years	Total number	One year	Five years
Upper third	158	13.3	2.3*	149	24.1	8.5*
Middle third	571	15.3	3.0***	527	25.2	7.7***
Lower third	529	19.2	5.7+++	454	28.0	11.6+++
Site unspecified	97	9.8	1.2	78	9.4	1.5

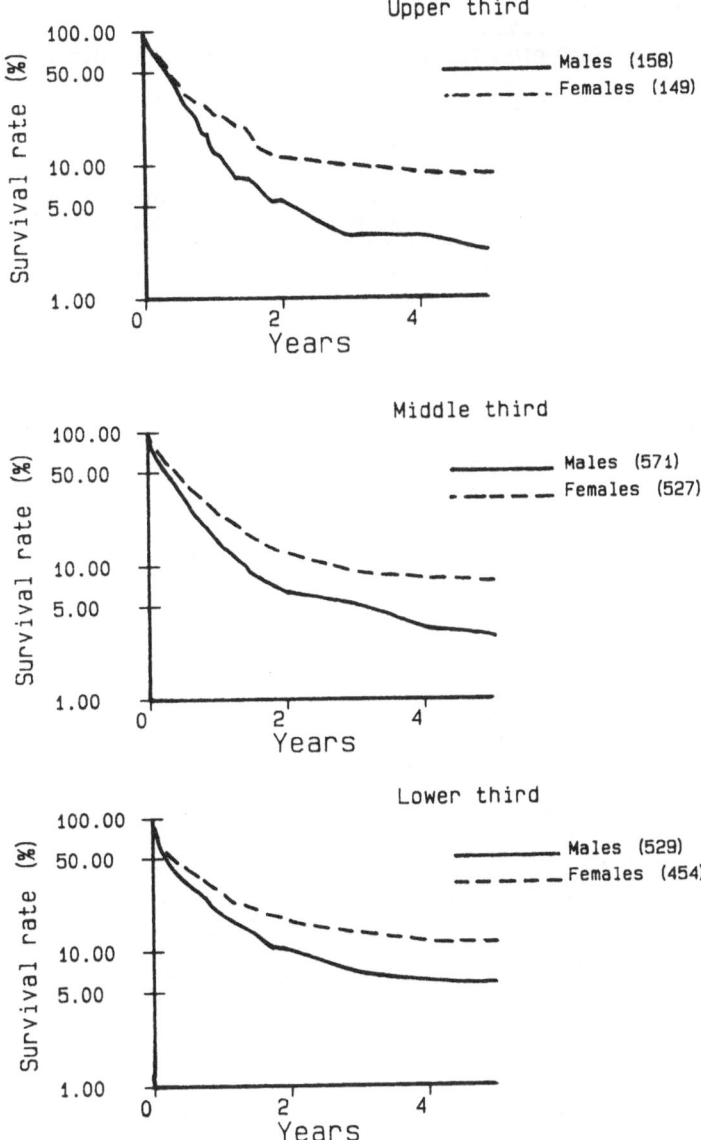

Figure 4.7 Squamous - Survival by Site and Sex.

Table 4.8

Only the middle and lower thirds are shown in the graphs, as there
were so few adenocarcinomas in the upper third.   The survival of
females was generally better but the differences were not significant.

Table 4.8   Adenocarcinoma.
            Age Adjusted Survival Rates (%) by Site and Sex.

	Males			Females		
	Total number	One year	Five year	Total number	One year	Five year
Upper third	3	0.0	0.0	6	18.0	0.0
Middle third	51	18.4	0.0	31	10.1	3.6
Lower third	130	17.6	0.0	51	16.4	2.4
Site unspecified	5	20.8	0.0	6	34.8	0.0

Middle third

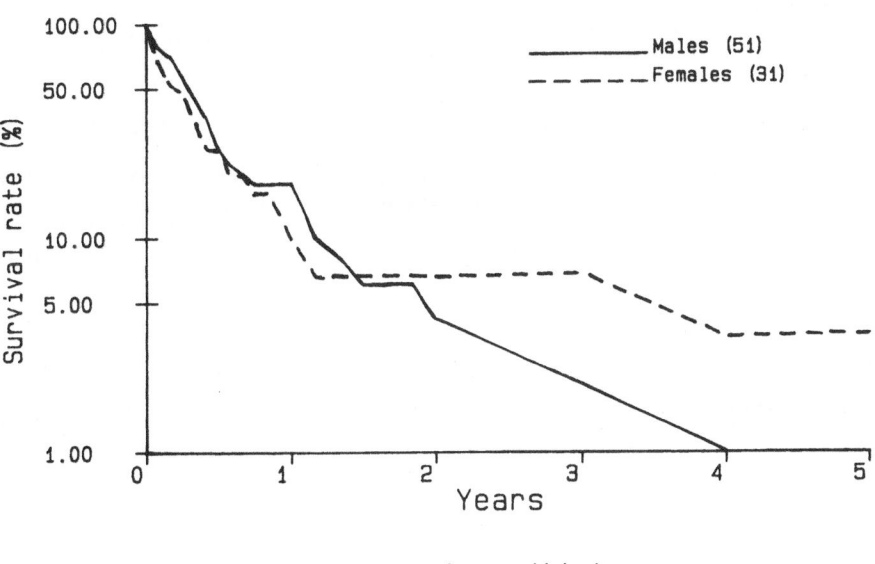

Lower third

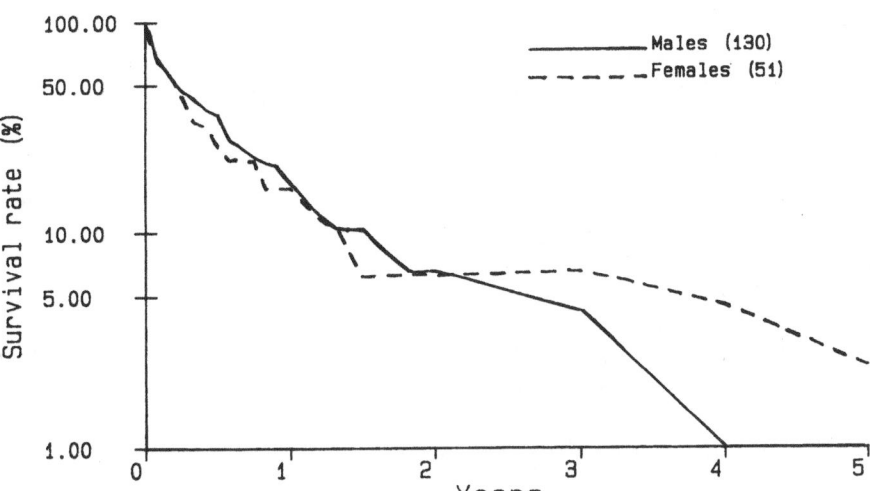

Figure 4.8   Adenocarcinoma - Survival by Site and Sex.

Table 4.9

The numbers of anaplastic tumours are too small for the differences to have any statistical significance.

Table 4.9   Anaplastic Carcinoma.
            Age Adjusted Survival Rates (%) by Site and Sex.

	Males			Females		
	Total number	One year	Five years	Total number	One year	Five years
Upper third	10	10.6	0.0	5	0.0	0.0
Middle third	58	12.7	0.0	52	6.0	2.2
Lower third	85	9.9	1.4	45	7.0	2.7
Site unspecified	8	0.0	0.0	8	13.2	0.0

Middle third

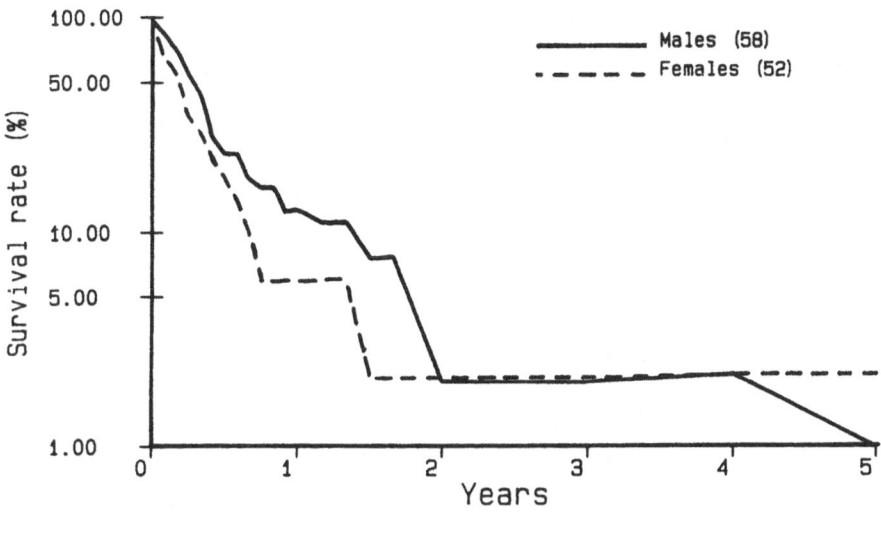

Lower third

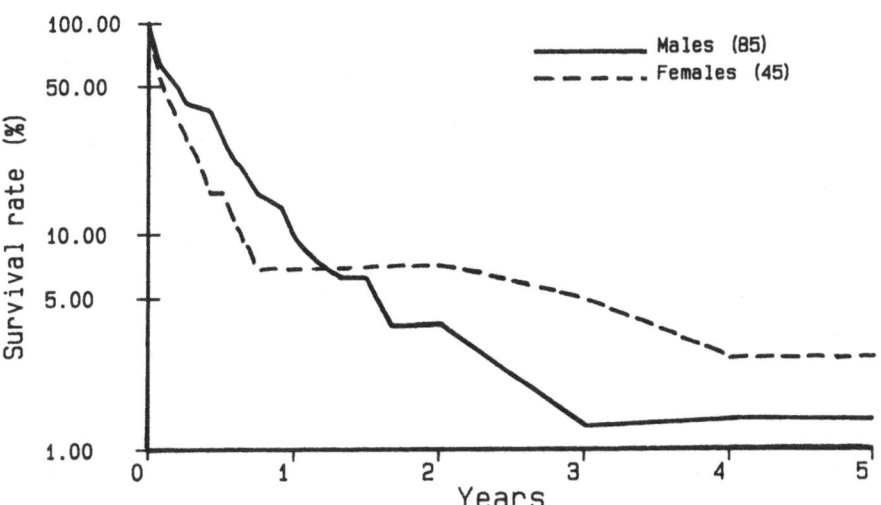

Figure 4.9   Anaplastic - Survival by Site and Sex.

Table 4.10

Survival at both 1 and 5 years is better for females than males at all ages, except for the 5-year survival in males under 40.

In these tables, and in Tables 4.11, 4.12 and 4.13, crude survival rates only are used. When broken down by age, the differences between crude and age-adjusted rates are negligible.

Table 4.10.1   Crude 1 Year Survival Rates by Age and Sex for 4680 Patients.

	Total		Males		Females	
	Number	(%)	Number	(%)	Number	(%)
20–24	1	0.0	1	0.0	0	–
25–29	2	50.0	2	50.0	0	–
30–34	16	31.2	6	33.3	10	30.0
35–39	28	50.0	15	46.7	13	53.8
40–44	71	26.8	31	25.8	40	27.5
45–49	186	16.7	90	8.9	96	24.0
50–54	314	21.7	174	17.2	140	27.1
55–59	499	20.8	299	17.1	200	26.5
60–64	637	16.5	402	14.4	235	20.0
65–69	744	13.0	457	10.5	287	17.1
70–74	801	12.9	457	9.6	344	17.2
75–79	667	8.2	367	7.4	300	9.3
80–84	447	5.6	207	4.8	240	6.2
85–89	208	3.4	89	3.4	119	3.4
90–94	54	0.0	21	0.0	33	0.0
95+	5	20.0	2	0.0	3	33.3

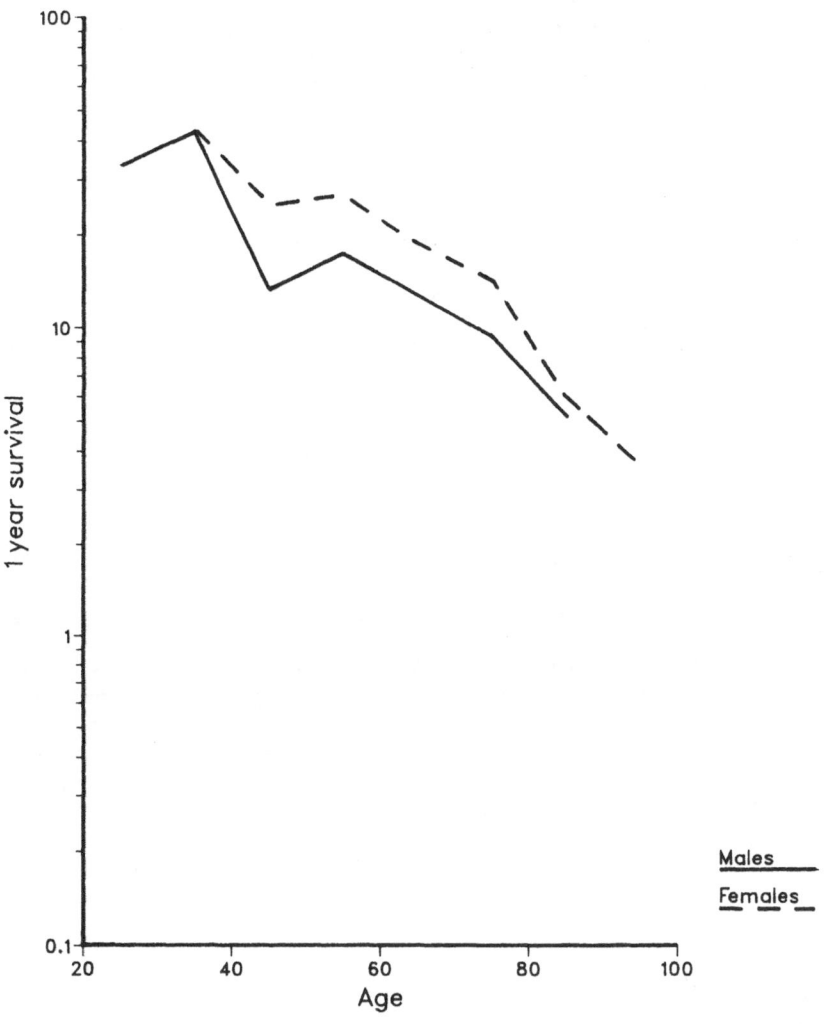

Figure 4.10.1   All Cases - 1-year Survival by Age and Sex.

Table 4.10.2   Crude 5 Year Survival Rates by Age and Sex for 4680
               Patients.

	Total		Males		Females	
	Number	(%)	Number	(%)	Number	(%)
20–24	1	0.0	1	0.0	0	–
25–29	2	50.0	2	50.0	0	–
30–34	16	0.0	6	0.0	10	0.0
35–39	28	17.9	15	26.7	13	7.7
40–44	71	12.7	31	12.9	40	12.5
45–49	186	3.8	90	0.0	96	7.3
50–54	314	6.7	174	5.2	140	8.6
55–59	499	6.2	299	2.7	200	11.5
60–64	637	3.9	402	2.2	235	6.8
65–69	744	3.4	457	1.5	287	6.3
70–74	801	2.4	457	0.7	344	4.7
75–79	667	0.4	367	0.3	300	0.7
80–84	447	0.4	207	0.0	240	0.8
85–89	208	0.0	89	0.0	119	0.0
90–94	54	0.0	21	0.0	33	0.0
95+	5	0.0	2	0.0	3	0.0

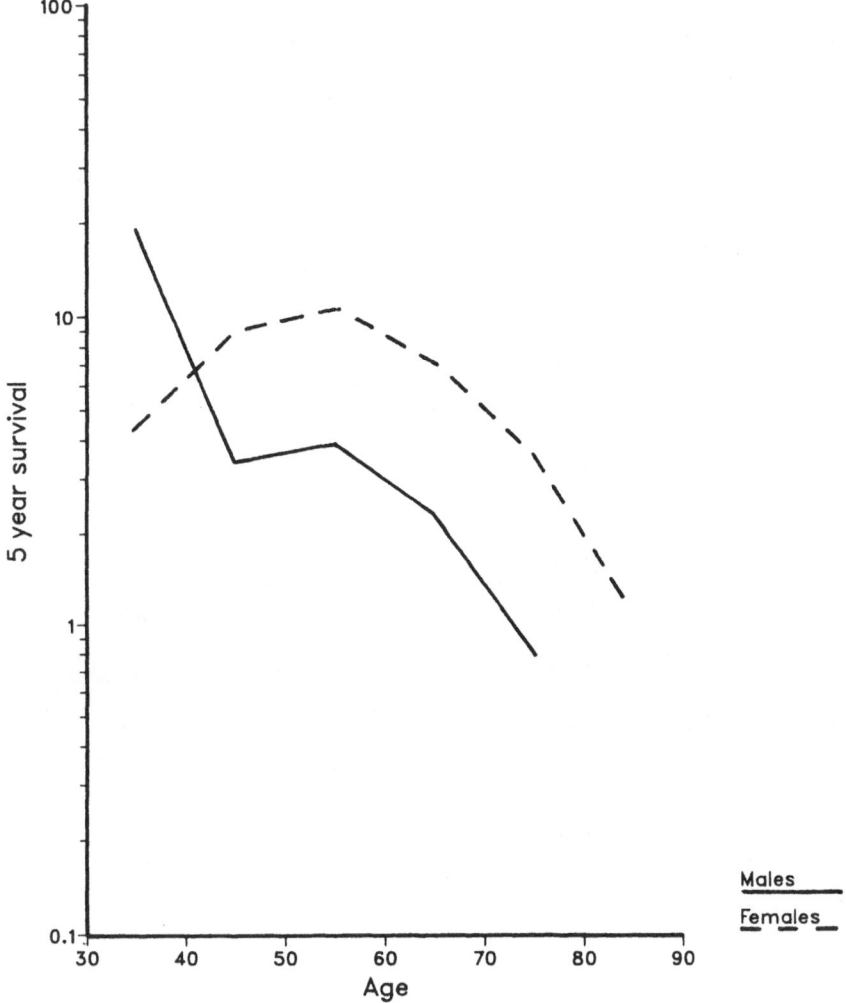

Figure 4.10.2   All Cases - 5-year Survival by Age and Sex.

Table 4.11

The majority of tumours are squamous so these results reflect those
for the whole population - shown in Table 4.10.

Table 4.11.1   Squamous Cell Carcinoma.
               Crude 1 Year Survival Rates by Age and Sex.

	Total		Males		Females	
	Number	(%)	Number	(%)	Number	(%)
20–24	1	0.0	1	0.0	0	–
25–29	2	50.0	2	50.0	0	–
30–34	13	30.8	4	25.0	9	33.3
35–39	24	54.2	12	50.0	12	58.3
40–44	48	33.3	17	35.3	31	32.3
45–49	130	20.8	52	7.7	78	29.5
50–54	227	28.2	111	24.3	116	31.9
55–59	348	24.7	192	18.7	156	32.1
60–64	408	20.3	244	16.4	164	26.2
65–69	444	17.8	253	13.8	191	23.0
70–74	438	18.7	236	14.0	202	24.3
75–79	290	12.8	148	10.8	142	14.8
80–84	127	6.3	60	5.0	67	7.5
85–89	51	5.9	18	5.6	33	6.1
90–94	11	0.0	4	0.0	7	0.0
95+	1	0.0	1	0.0	0	–

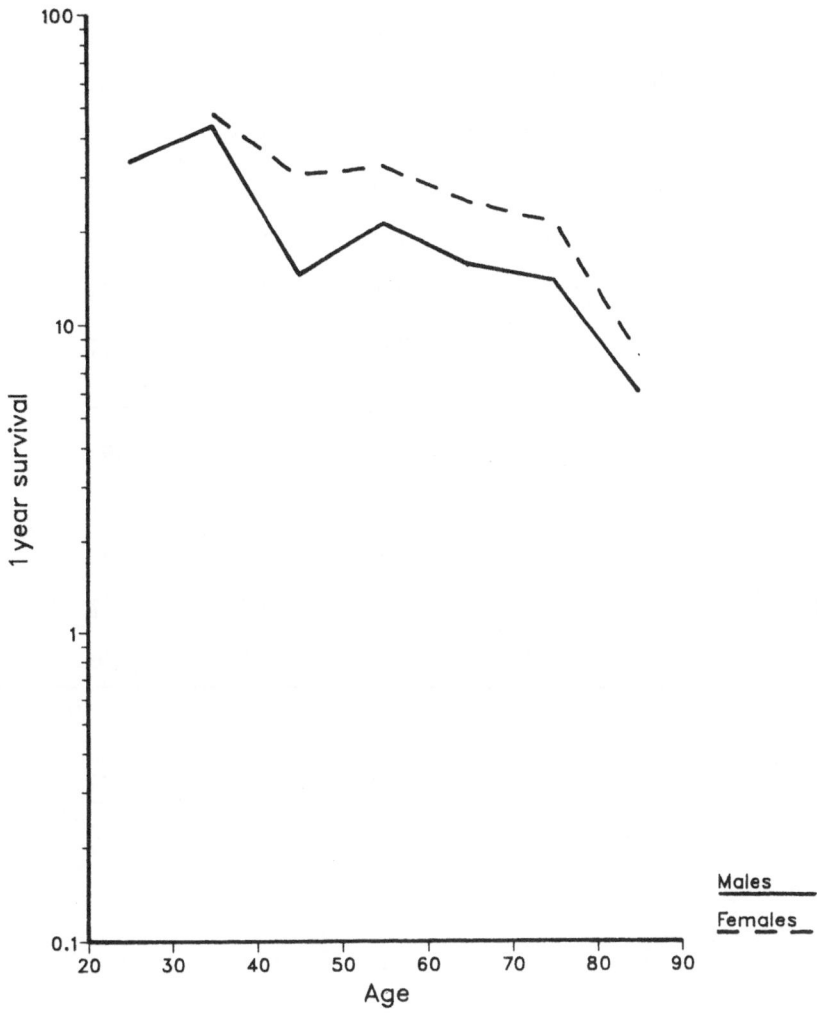

Figure 4.11.1   Squamous - 1-year Survival by Age and Sex.

Table 4.11.2   Squamous Cell Carcinoma.
              Crude 5 Year Survival Rates by Age and Sex.

	Total Number	Total (%)	Males Number	Males (%)	Females Number	Females (%)
20–24	1	0.0	1	0.0	0	–
25–29	2	50.0	2	50.0	0	–
30–34	13	0.0	4	0.0	9	0.0
35–39	24	16.7	12	25.0	12	8.3
40–44	48	18.7	17	23.5	31	16.1
45–49	130	5.4	52	0.0	78	9.0
50–54	227	8.8	111	8.1	116	9.5
55–59	348	8.3	192	4.2	156	13.5
60–64	408	5.4	244	2.9	164	9.1
65–69	444	5.4	253	2.8	191	8.9
70–74	438	4.3	236	1.3	202	7.9
75–79	290	1.0	148	0.7	142	1.4
80–84	127	0.0	60	0.0	67	0.0
85–89	51	0.0	18	0.0	33	0.0
90–94	11	0.0	4	0.0	7	0.0
95+	1	0.0	1	0.0	0	–

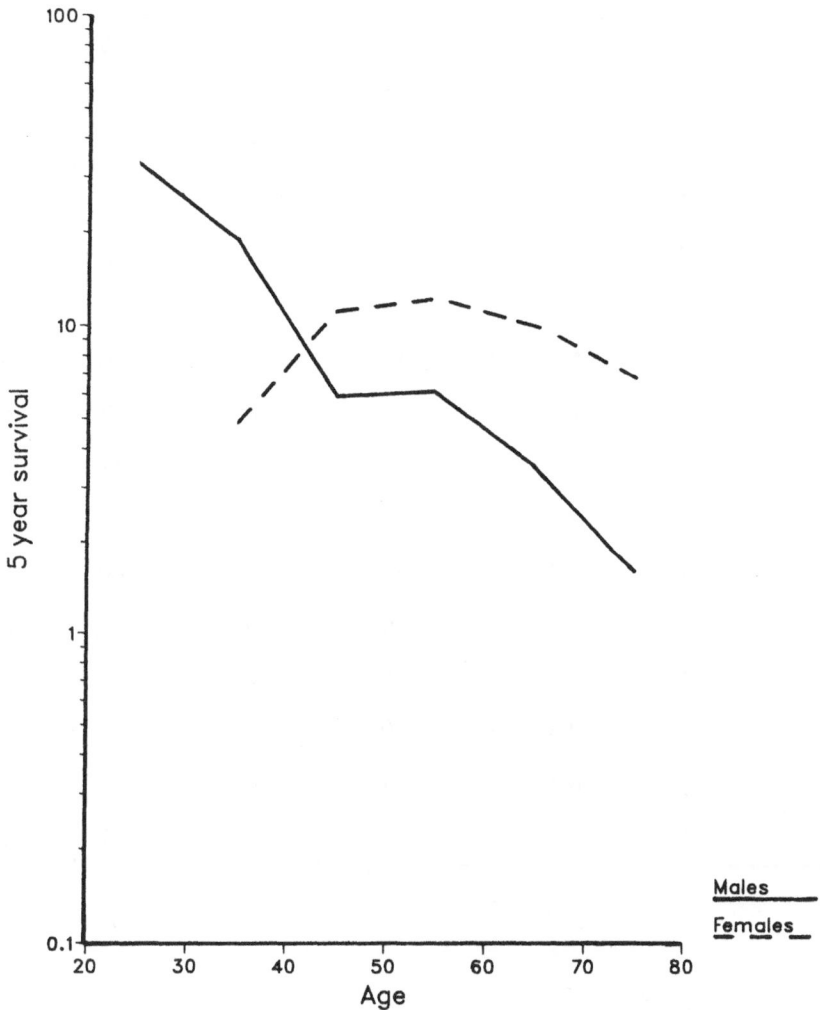

Figure 4.11.2   Squamous - 5-year Survival by Age and Sex.

Table 4.12

Clearly there is no significant difference in survival at 1 year
between the sexes at different age groups for adenocarcinomas.
Only two cases (both female, aged 50-59) were alive at 5 years.

Table 4.12   Adenocarcinoma.
             Crude 1 Year Survival Rates by Age and Sex.

| | Total | | Males | | Females | |
	Number	(%)	Number	(%)	Number	(%)
20-24	0	-	0	-	0	-
25-29	0	-	0	-	0	-
30-34	1	100.0	1	100.0	0	-
35-39	2	0.0	1	0.0	1	0.0
40-44	7	14.3	5	0.0	2	50.0
45-49	14	28.6	13	30.8	1	0.0
50-54	26	11.5	21	9.5	5	20.0
55-59	29	27.6	22	31.8	7	14.3
60-64	49	26.5	38	28.9	11	18.2
65-69	49	14.3	35	11.4	14	21.4
70-74	47	12.8	27	11.1	20	15.0
75-79	40	5.0	20	0.0	20	10.0
80-84	14	7.1	5	0.0	9	11.1
85-89	2	0.0	0	-	2	0.0
90-94	3	0.0	1	0.0	2	0.0
95+	0	-	0	-	0	-

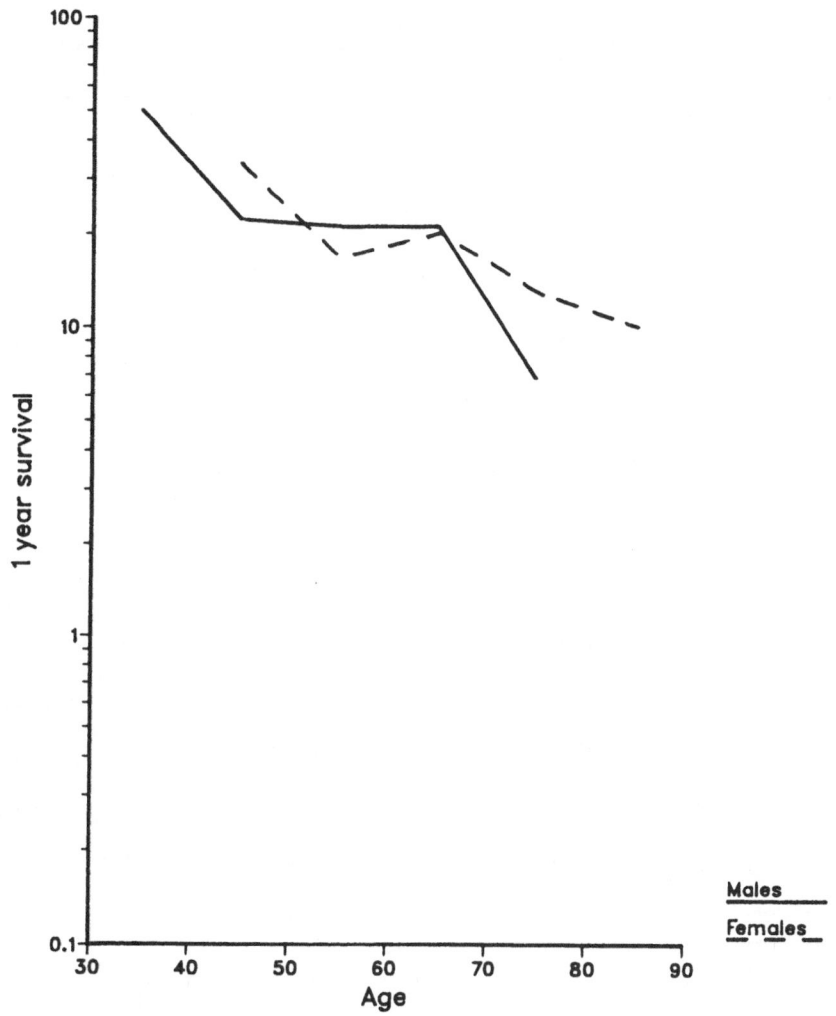

Figure 4.12   Adenocarcinoma — 1-year Survival by Age and Sex.
              (Data from Table 4.12 plotted as 10 year age groups.)

Table 4.13

The numbers of cases of anaplastic carcinoma, when broken down by age, are too small to demonstrate survival differences between the sexes at 1 year.   Only one male and two females (all aged 60-69) were alive at 5 years.

Table 4.13   Anaplastic Carcinoma.
             Crude 1 Year Survival Rates by Age and Sex.

| | Total | | Males | | Females | |
	Number	(%)	Number	(%)	Number	(%)
20-24	0	-	0	-	0	-
25-29	0	-	0	-	0	-
30-34	1	0.0	0	-	1	0.0
35-39	0	-	0	-	0	-
40-44	4	25.0	2	50.0	2	0.0
45-49	12	0.0	8	0.0	4	0.0
50-54	22	4.5	16	6.2	6	0.0
55-59	29	6.9	18	11.1	11	0.0
60-64	34	14.7	26	15.4	8	12.5
65-69	63	7.9	39	7.7	24	8.3
70-74	44	6.8	22	9.1	22	4.5
75-79	33	15.2	19	10.5	14	21.4
80-84	19	5.3	8	12.5	11	0.0
85-89	9	0.0	3	0.0	6	0.0
90-94	1	0.0	0	-	1	0.0
95+	0	-	0	-	0	-

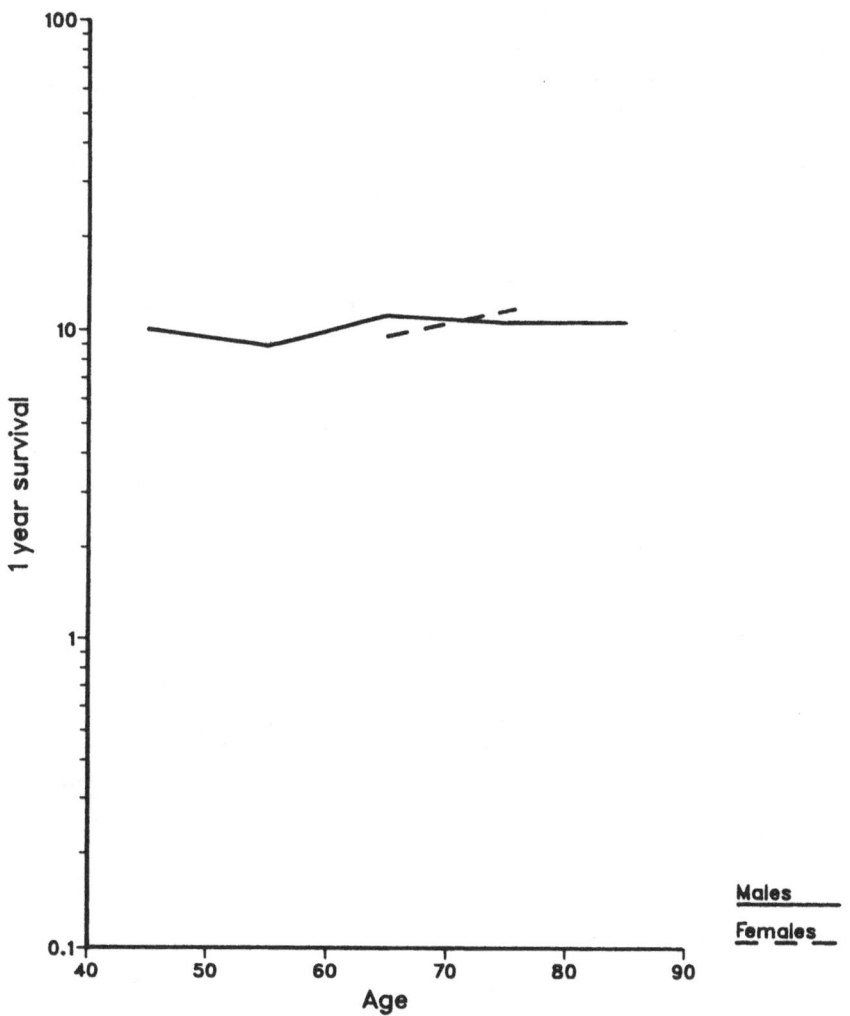

Figure 4.13   Anaplastic — 1-year Survival by Age and Sex.
(Data from Table 4.13 plotted as 10 year age groups.)

Tables 4.14, 4.15 and 4.16

If the first quinquennium is excluded, then survival rates over the next 15-year period show no significant improvement generally, or within sexes or sites.

Table 4.14   Annual Age Adjusted Survival Rates by Quinquennium for 4680 Patients.

Quinquennium	Total number	% survival in years				
		1	2	3	4	5
1957 - 61	862	12.6	6.4	4.9	3.5	3.5
1962 - 66	1169	13.6	6.1	5.2	4.0	3.5
1967 - 71	1209	14.3	7.5	5.3	4.7	4.5
1972 - 76	1440	16.0	7.5	4.9	3.8	3.6

Table 4.15   Annual Age Adjusted Survival Rates by Quinquennium
             and Sex for 4680 Patients.

Quinquennium		Total number	% survival in years				
			1	2	3	4	5
1957 - 61	M	500	11.4	5.9	4.1	2.3	2.1
	F	362	14.1	7.0	5.9	5.1	5.2
1962 - 66	M	662	10.6	3.4	2.6	1.8	1.1
	F	507	17.4	9.6	8.3	6.8	6.5
1967 - 71	M	661	12.5	5.5	3.5	2.7	2.6
	F	548	16.4	9.8	7.4	7.0	6.7
1972 - 76	M	797	13.2	5.7	3.5	3.0	2.8
	F	643	19.4	9.6	6.5	4.8	4.6

Table 4.16   Age Adjusted Five Year Survival Rates (%) by
             Quinquennium and Site for 4680 Patients.

Quinquennium	Site:			
	Upper third	Middle third	Lower third	Site unspecified
1957 - 61	1.3 (81)	3.6 (288)	4.9 (322)	1.4 (171)
1962 - 66	3.6 (138)	4.1 (376)	4.2 (489)	0.0 (166)
1967 - 71	6.0 (120)	2.8 (455)	6.4 (528)	0.0 (106)
1972 - 76	6.2 (120)	4.0 (573)	3.6 (588)	0.0 (159)

5

Treatment

In the treatment of oesophageal carcinoma many different methods are used and in the individual patient these may be combined, either at the time of initial diagnosis, or subsequently. Therefore in order to simplify the situation this analysis is confined to the treatment given at the time of first presentation and the main groups have been defined according to what the treatment was intended to achieve. Patients who had therapy which was intended to diminish or eliminate the activity of the primary lesion (e.g. resection, radiotherapy, chemotherapy) form the *'primary anti-tumour treatment'* group, while the rest constitute the *'no primary anti-tumour treatment'* group, consisting of patients who had intubation or by-pass for dysphagia, exploratory surgery or treatment directed only at metastases, together with those who had no initial treatment at all.

The data presented relates to the 4680 cases registered from 1957 to 1976 in order to correspond with the 5-year survival after treatment which is analysed in Chapter 6. All cases are analysed for treatment in relation to the histology and site of the tumour, and the age and sex of the patient. The primary anti-tumour treatment group (1911 patients) is then further analysed according to whether the treatment of the primary lesion was meant to be curative or palliative, by histology, site and sex.

5.1 SUMMARY OF FINDINGS

At the time of presentation only 40.8% of patients had any treatment which was expected to restrict the growth of the primary tumour, and when such treatment was given it was intended to be curative in only 68.1% of those cases. Surgical resection was the most commonly used form of anti-tumour treatment and was applied to all histological types, but mainly in the middle and lower thirds of the oesophagus. Radiotherapy was used mainly for squamous carcinomas (particularly of the upper third) and anaplastic tumours. Treatment was intended to be curative more often when surgical resection was used, in tumours of the lower third, and in females. Conversely, treatment

92

was intended to be palliative more often with radiotherapy, tumours of the middle and upper thirds and anaplastic carcinomas. Chemotherapy was never used with curative intent.

Table 5.1

Of the 4680 patients only 1911 (40.8%) had treatment which was intended to restrict the growth of the primary tumour. The other 2769 patients (59.2%) had either no treatment (presumably due to age, advanced disease or poor general condition), exploratory surgery or symptomatic treatment alone (usually for dysphagia). Anti-tumour treatment consisted of surgical resection (± additional therapy) in 24.4% of the whole population and radiotherapy and/or chemotherapy in 16.4%.

Table 5.1 Type of Treatment: Distribution.

	No. of patients	%
Primary anti-tumour treatment		
Resection (±RT/CT) (24.4%)		
Resection only	1104	23.6
Resection + radiotherapy	29	0.6
Resection + chemotherapy	8	0.2
Resection + radiotherapy + chemotherapy	2	0.1
Radiotherapy/Chemotherapy (± surgery other than resection) (16.4%)		
Radiotherapy	725	15.5
Chemotherapy	31	0.7
Radiotherapy + chemotherapy	12	0.2
No primary anti-tumour treatment		
Other treatment (25.4%)		
By-pass	60	1.3
Insertion of tube + exploratory surgery	479	10.2
Insertion of tube only	523	11.2
Exploratory surgery only	120	2.5
Treatment to metastases (Surgery or R/T)	6	0.1
No treatment (33.8%)	1581	33.8
TOTAL	4680	100.0

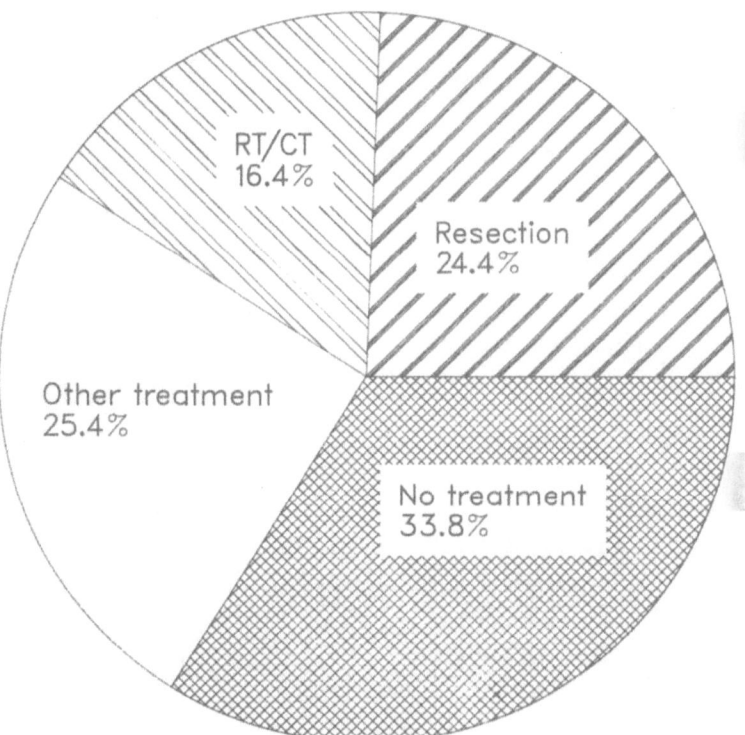

Figure 5.1   Type of Treatment: Distribution.

Table 5.2

Anti-tumour treatment was given in 58.9% of squamous carcinomas, compared with 45.2% of adenocarcinomas and 43.2% of anaplastic tumours; these differences are very highly significant. Resection was used equally in squamous carcinomas and adenocarcinomas, but radiotherapy and chemotherapy were used mainly in squamous and anaplastic carcinomas. The 'other histology' group comprises patients with histology 'not specified' or 'suggestive of malignancy' (see Chapter 3) and these are excluded from Figure 5.2 as the numbers are small. The low rate of anti-tumour treatment (9.3%) in the 'no histology' group reflects the advanced nature of the disease in this category.

Table 5.2 Type of Treatment: Distribution by Histological Category.

	Squamous cell ca.		Adenoca.		Anaplastic		Other		No histology	
	No.	%	No.	%	No.	%	No.	%	No.	%
Primary anti-tumour treatment										
Resection (± RT/CT)	955	37.3	106	37.4	60	22.2	7	10.9	15	1.0
Radiotherapy/Chemotherapy (± other surgery)	555	21.6	22	7.8	57	21.0	10	15.6	124	8.3
No primary anti-tumour treatment										
Other treatment	605	23.6	94	33.2	94	34.7	15	23.5	380	25.3
No treatment	448	17.5	61	21.6	60	22.1	32	50.0	980	65.4
TOTAL	2563	100.0	283	100.0	271	100.0	64	100.0	1499	100.0

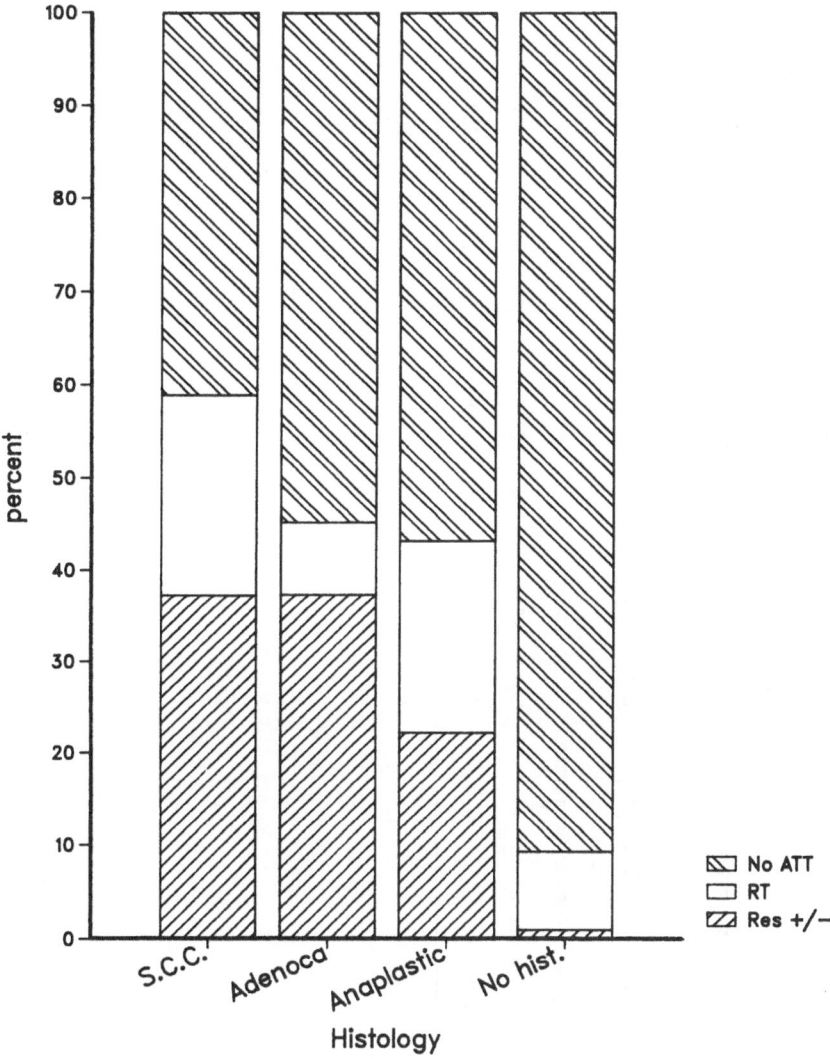

Figure 5.2   Treatment by Histological Category.

Table 5.3

When divided by site, anti-tumour treatment was used in 55.3% of tumours in the upper third, compared with 48.1% in the middle third (highly significant) and 39.9% in the lower third (very highly significant). The type of treatment used, however, varied inversely. Most of the proximal tumours were treated by radiotherapy, while most the distal tumours were treated by resection.

Table 5.3   Type of Treatment: Distribution by Site.

	Upper third No.	%	Middle third No.	%	Lower third No.	%	Unspecified No.	%
Primary anti-tumour treatment								
Resection (± RT/CT)	46	10.0	423	25.0	633	32.8	41	6.8
Radiotherapy/Chemotherapy	208	45.3	391	23.1	136	7.1	33	5.5
No primary anti-tumour treatment								
Other treatment	69	15.0	472	27.9	533	27.7	114	18.9
No treatment	136	29.7	406	24.0	625	32.4	414	68.8
TOTAL	459	100.0	1692	100.0	1927	100.0	602	100.0

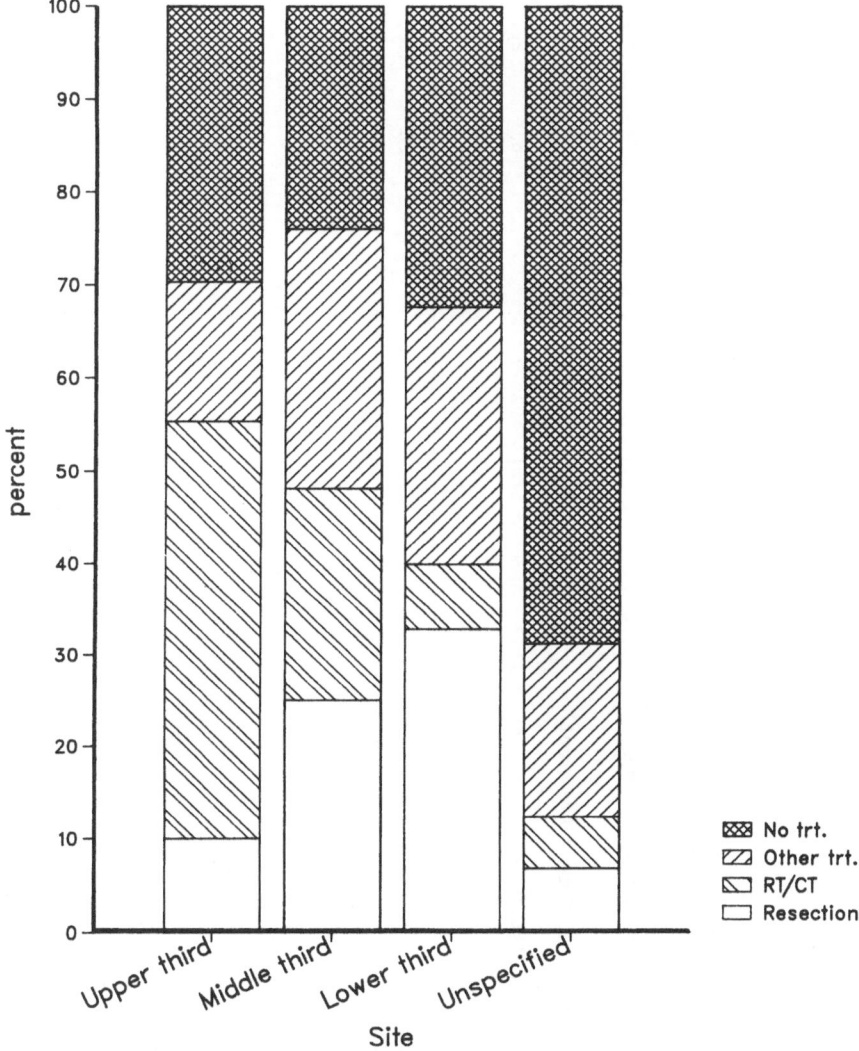

Figure 5.3   Treatment by Site.

Table 5.4

Anti-tumour treatment was used in 39.1% of males compared with 43.0% of females; this difference is highly significant. More important, however, is the finding that resection was performed in only 21.5% of males compared with 28.1% of females; this difference is also highly significant and may contribute to the improved survival in females noted in Chapter 4.

Table 5.4 Type of Treatment: Distribution by Sex.

	Males		Females	
	No.	%	No.	%
Primary anti-tumour treatment				
Resection	564	21.5**	579	28.1**
Radiotherapy/Chemotherapy	460	17.6*	308	14.9*
No primary anti-tumour treatment				
Other treatment	721	27.5	467	22.7
No treatment	875	33.4	706	34.3
TOTAL	2620	100.0	2060	100.0

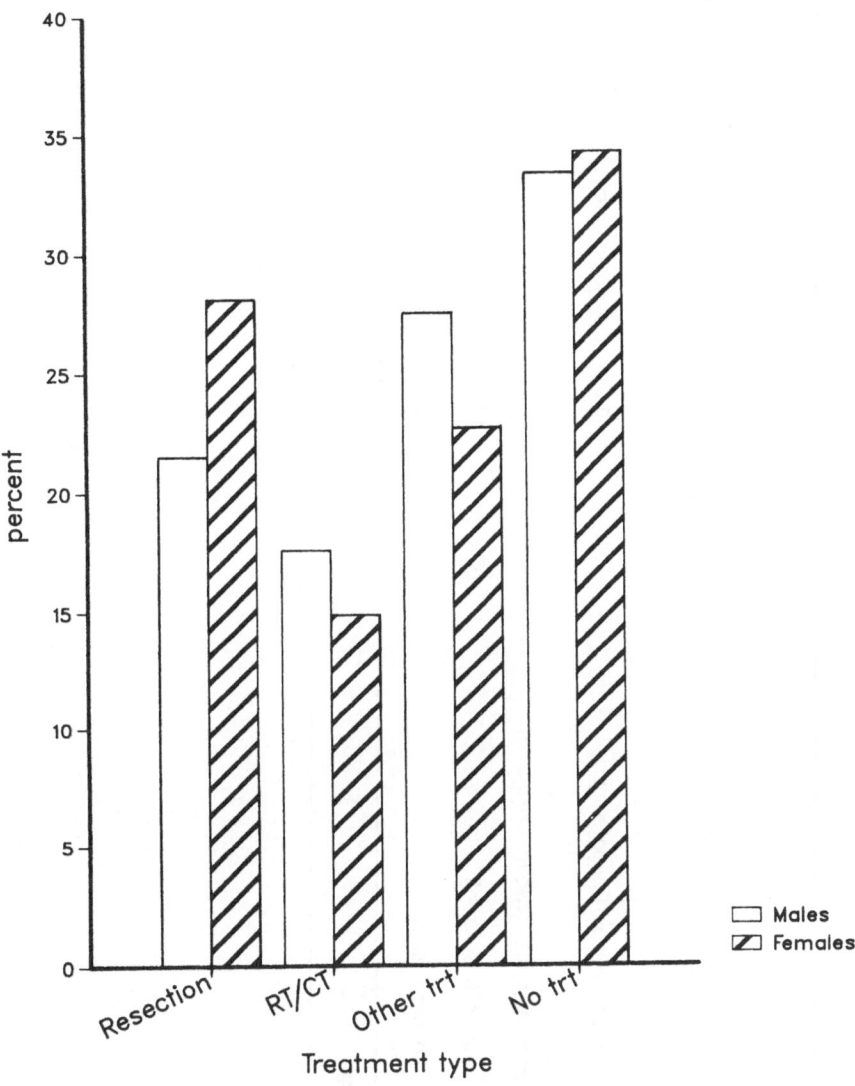

Figure 5.4   Treatment by Sex.

Table 5.5

The mean age of the resected females was 1.5 years younger than for resected males, but it seems unlikely that this difference alone is sufficient to account for the increased female resection rate noted in Table 5.4.

Table 5.5 Type of Treatment: Mean Age by Sex.

	MALES		FEMALES	
	Mean age	Standard deviation	Mean age	Standard deviation
Primary anti-tumour treatment				
Resection	62.5	9.2	61.9	10.0
Radiotherapy/Chemotherapy	65.4	11.0	65.4	12.0
No primary anti-tumour treatment				
Other treatment	67.9	10.6	69.9	11.8
No treatment	72.1	10.0	75.3	10.4
TOTAL	67.7	10.8	68.8	12.2

.

Table 5.6

In the 1911 patients who received anti-tumour treatment the intention was curative in 68.1% and palliative in 31.9%. The curative rate for resection, however, was 83.0% compared with 48.4% for radiotherapy. Chemotherapy was never used with a curative intent.

Table 5.6 Primary Anti-tumour Treatment: Curative v Palliative.

	Curative No.	%	Palliative No.	%	Total No.	%
Resection (± RT/CT)						
Resection only	919	83.2	185	16.8	1104	100.0
Resection + R/T	23	79.3	6	20.7	29	100.0
Resection + C/T	6	75.0	2	25.0	8	100.0
Resection + R/T + C/T	1	50.0	1	50.0	2	100.0
Radiotherapy/Chemotherapy (no resection)						
Radiotherapy	351	48.4	374	51.6	725	100.0
Chemotherapy	0	0.0	31	100.0	31	100.0
Radiotherapy + chemotherapy	2	16.7	10	83.3	12	100.0
Total anti-tumour treatment	1302	68.1	609	31.9	1911	100.0

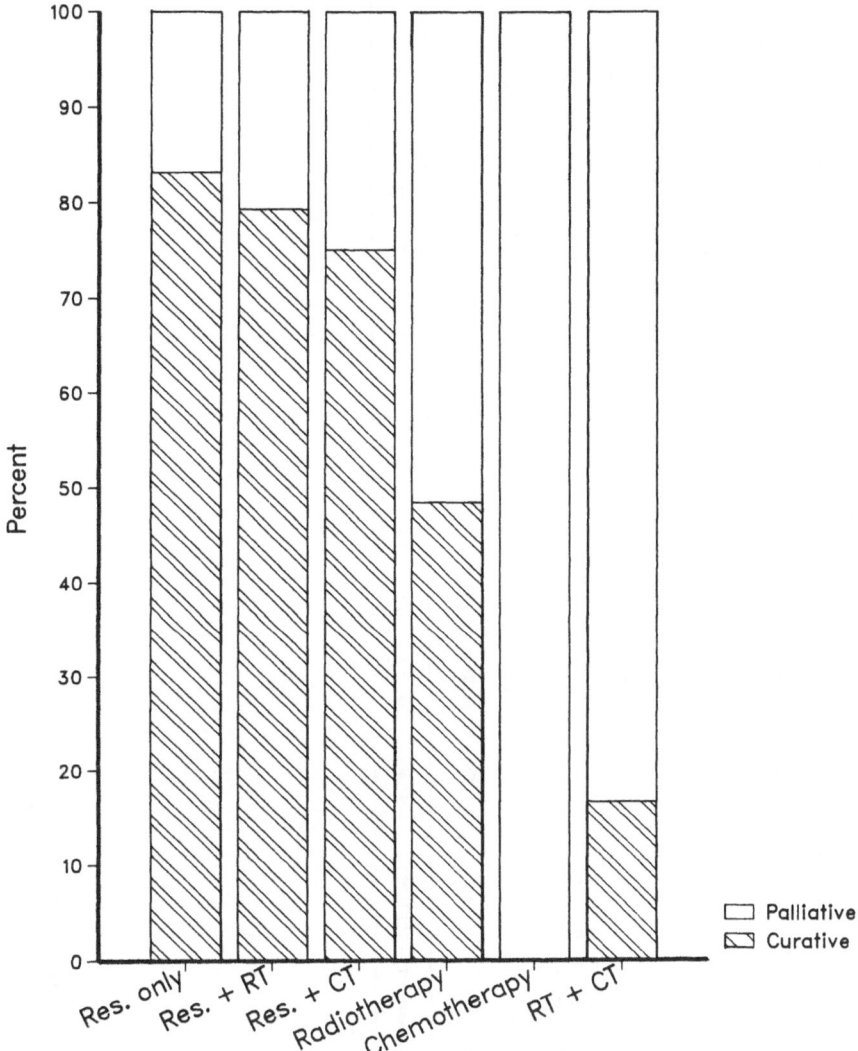

Figure 5.6   Primary Anti-tumour Treatment (PATT): Curative v.
Palliative.

Table 5.7

Anti-tumour treatment was intended to be curative in only 54.7% of anaplastic tumours, but in 72.2% of squamous tumours (very highly significant) and in 71.9% of adenocarcinomas (highly significant). The 'other histology' group is omitted from Figure 5.7 as the numbers are small.

Table 5.7 Primary Anti-tumour Treatment: Curative v Palliative by Histological Category.

	Squamous cell ca. No.	%	Adenoca. No.	%	Anaplastic No.	%	Other histology No.	%	No histology No.	%
Resection ($\pm$ RT/CT)										
Curative	806	53.4	86	67.2	40	34.2	6	35.3	11	7.9
Palliative	149	9.9	20	15.6	20	17.1	1	5.9	4	2.9
Radiotherapy/Chemotherapy (no resection)										
Curative	284	18.8	6	4.7	24	20.5	3	17.6	36	25.9
Palliative	271	17.9	16	12.5	33	28.2	7	41.2	88	63.3
Total anti-tumour treatment	1510	100.0	128	100.0	117	100.0	17	100.0	139	100.0

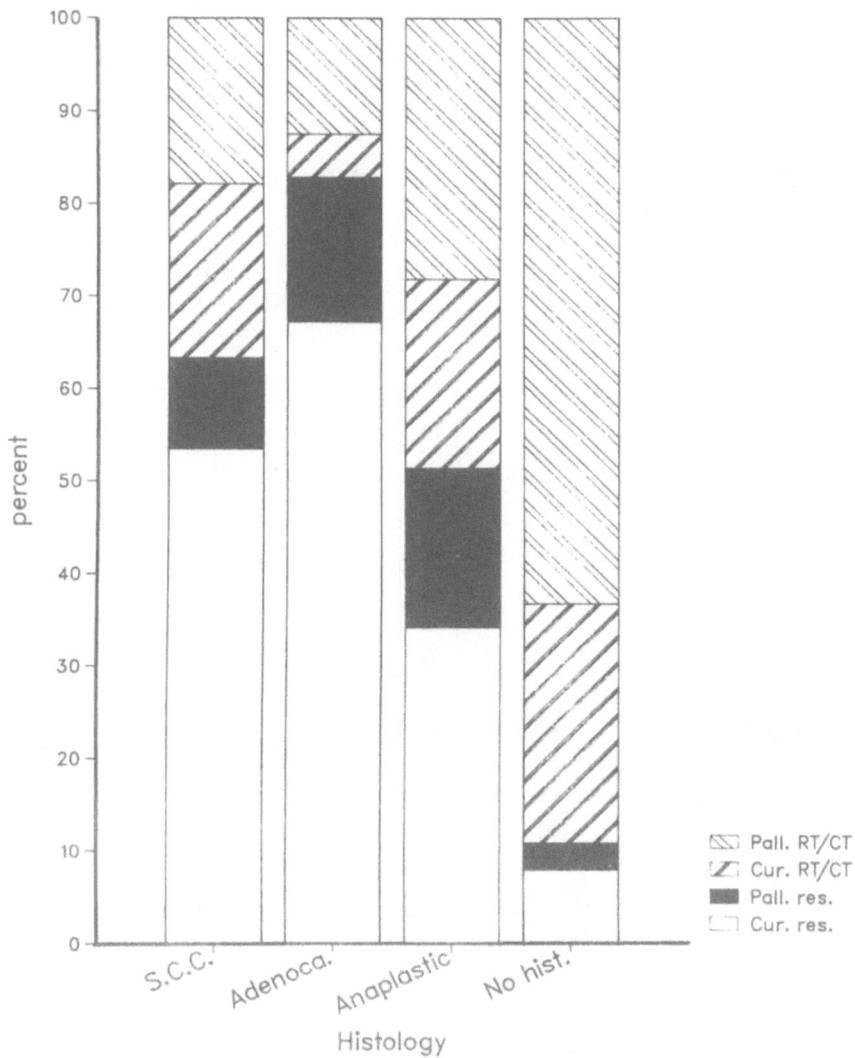

Figure 5.7   PATT: Curative v. Palliative by Histology.

Table 5.8

When divided by site, anti-tumour treatment was intended to be curative in 64.6% in the upper third and 64.5% in the middle third, compared with 73.7% in the lower third. These figures simply reflect the fact that resection was used more often in the lower third (see Table 5.3) and was more often intended to be curative (see Table 5.6).

Table 5.8 Primary Anti-tumour Treatment: Curative v Palliative by Site.

	Upper third No.	%	Middle third No.	%	Lower third No.	%	Site unspecified No.	%
Resection								
Curative	38	15.0	355	43.6	520	67.6	36	48.6
Palliative	8	3.1	68	8.4	113	14.7	5	6.8
Radiotherapy/Chemotherapy								
Curative	126	49.6	170	20.9	47	6.1	10	13.5
Palliative	82	32.3	221	27.1	89	11.6	23	31.1
Total anti-tumour treatments	254	100.0	814	100.0	769	100.0	74	100.0

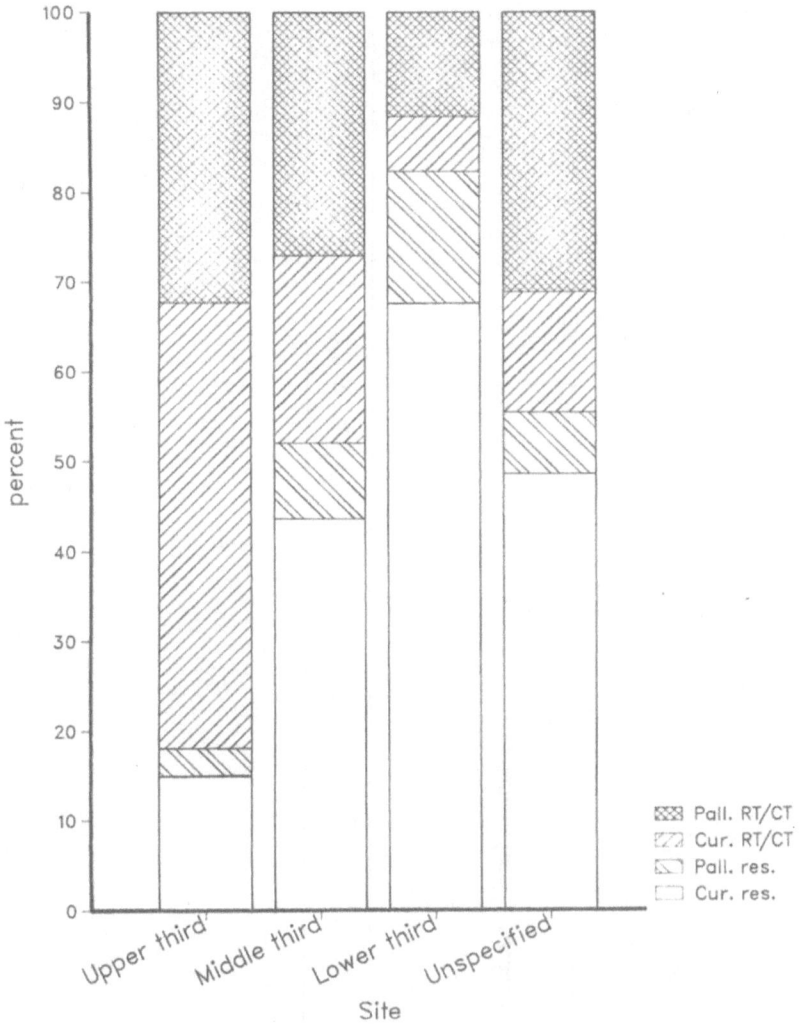

Figure 5.8   PATT: Curative v. Palliative by Site.

Table 5.9

Anti-tumour treatment was intended to be curative in 64.5% of males, compared with 71.3% of females; this difference is highly significant. When curative resection alone is considered, the difference between the sexes is even greater and is very highly significant.

Table 5.9 Primary Anti-tumour Treatment: Curative v Palliative by Sex.

	Males No.	Males %	Females No.	Females %
Resection				
Curative	456	44.5***	493	55.6***
Palliative	108	10.6	86	9.7
Radiotherapy/Chemotherapy				
Curative	214	20.9	139	15.7
Palliative	246	24.0	169	19.0
Total primary anti-tumour treatments	1024	100.0	887	100.0

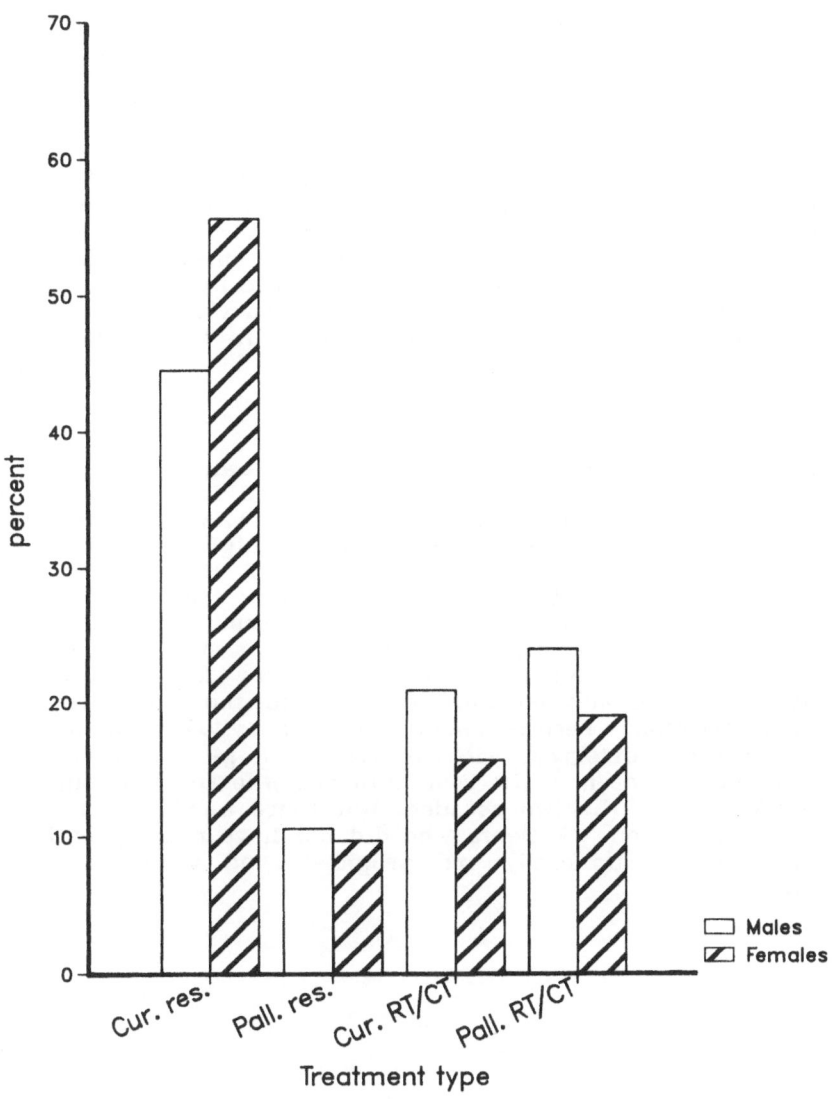

Figure 5.9   PATT: Curative v. Palliative by Sex.

6

Survival after Treatment

Data in this chapter relates to the same 4680 cases and treatment groups which have been defined in Chapter 5. Most of the analysis is concerned with patients who received primary anti-tumour treatment and detailed survival data is given for curative and palliative treatments, and surgical resection specifically, by sex, site, histology, node status and age. Two-year survival data for the no primary anti-tumour treatment group is given in Table 6.15.

6.1 SUMMARY OF FINDINGS

In general the results reflect the poor overall survival noted in Chapter 4, but 5-year survival was achieved in 7.7% of all cases having primary anti-tumour treatment and in 11.1% of patients having curative treatments. Five-year survival was highest in patients with node-negative squamous tumours treated by resection, but some patients with node-positive squamous tumours treated by resection survived to 5 years, even when operation was thought to be palliative. Radiotherapy also produced some 5-year survivors in patients with squamous and anaplastic tumours. Very few adenocarcinomas survived 5 years and all were confined to the group treated by curative resection. Females showed better survival rates than males, irrespective of histology, site or treatment given. A significant improvement was seen in the results of radiotherapy (for upper-third tumours) between the two decades, but there was no change in the results of resection. Patients who did not have primary anti-tumour treatment had a uniformly bad prognosis and very few survived beyond 2 years.

Table 6.1

Of all the patients who had primary anti-tumour treatment, 28.2%
were alive at 1 year and 7.7% were alive at 5 years.   Long-term
survival was better with resection than with radiotherapy, but radiotherapy was much more often intended to be palliative (see Table
5.6).   The best results were seen when resection was combined with
radiotherapy or chemotherapy, but the numbers in these groups
were too small for the improvement to be significant.   Survival of
the no primary anti-tumour treatment group is given in greater
detail in Table 6.15; the lone 5-year survivor in this group did not
have a histological diagnosis but was not excluded by any of the
criteria used in this study (see Chapter 1, Section 1.2).

Table 6.1.1 One Year Crude and Age Adjusted Rates by Type of Treatment.

	Total number	No. alive	Crude rate (%)	Age adjusted rate (%)
Primary anti-tumour treatment				
[a] **Resection (± RT/CT)**	1143	411	36.0	36.9
Resection only	1104	395	35.8	36.8
Resection + radiotherapy	29	10	34.5	35.4
Resection + chemotherapy	8	5	62.5	63.6
Resection + radiotherapy + chemotherapy	2	1	50.0	50.2
[b] **Radiotherapy/Chemotherapy (no resection)**	768	127	16.5	17.3
Radiotherapy alone	725	127	17.5	18.3
Chemotherapy alone	31	0	0.0	0.0
Radiotherapy + chemotherapy	12	0	0.0	0.0
No primary anti-tumour treatment				
[c] **Other treatment**	1188	37	3.1	3.3
By-pass	60	2	3.3	3.5
Insertion of tube + exploratory surgery	479	10	2.1	2.2
Insertion of tube only	523	21	4.0	4.3
Exploratory surgery	120	3	2.5	2.6
Treatment to metastases (surgery or R/T)	6	1	16.7	17.2
[d] **No treatment**	1581	60	3.8	4.1
TOTAL	4680	635	13.6	14.3

Note : Letters in square brackets refer to lines on Figure 6.1.

Table 6.1.2 Five Year Crude and Age Adjusted Survival Rates by Type of Treatment.

	Total number	No. alive	Crude rate (%)	Age adjusted rate (%)
Primary anti-tumour treatment				
[a] **Resection (± RT/CT)**	1143	127	11.1	12.6
Resection only	1104	122	11.1	12.5
Resection + radiotherapy	29	4	13.8	15.4
Resection + chemotherapy	8	1	12.5	14.5
Resection + radiotherapy + chemotherapy	2	0	0.0	0.0
[b] **Radiotherapy/Chemotherapy (no resection)**	768	20	2.6	3.2
Radiotherapy alone	725	20	2.8	3.4
Chemotherapy alone	31	0	0.0	0.0
Radiotherapy + chemotherapy	12	0	0.0	0.0
No primary anti-tumour treatment				
[c] **Other treatment**	1188	0	0.0	0.0
By-pass	60	0	0.0	0.0
Insertion of tube + exploratory surgery	479	0	0.0	0.0
Insertion of tube only	523	0	0.0	0.0
Exploratory surgery	120	0	0.0	0.0
Treatment to metastases (surgery or R/T)	6	0	0.0	0.0
[d] **No treatment**	1581	1	0.1	0.1
TOTAL	4680	148	3.2	3.8

Note : Letters in square brackets refer to lines on Figure 6.1.

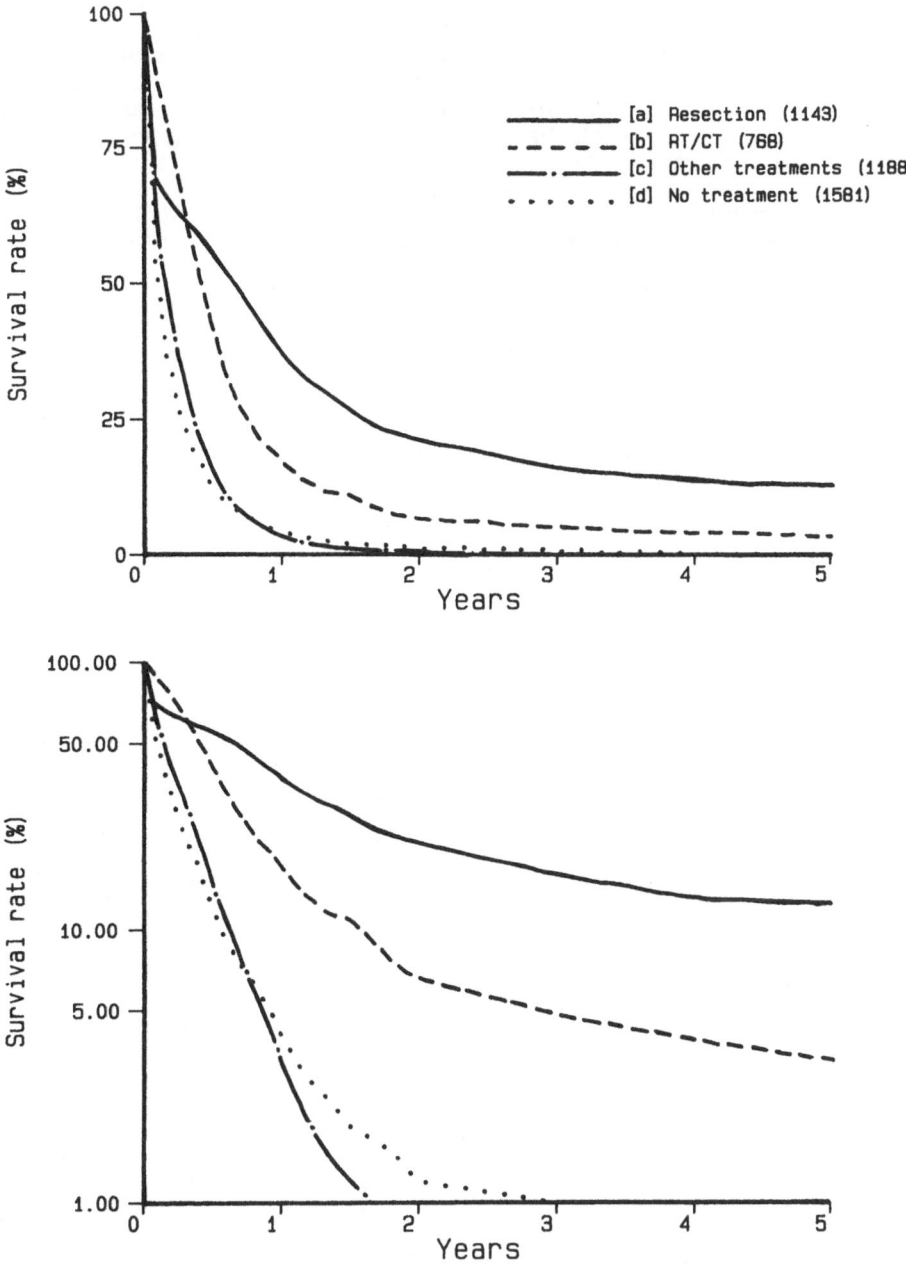

Figure 6.1   Annual Rate by Treatment.

Table 6.2

This shows that death within 1 month of the commencement of treatment is not confined to resected cases, although it is certainly highest in this group. Radiotherapy and chemotherapy, alone or in combination, had a 1-month mortality of at least 10%, though this is rarely mentioned when treatment options are being considered. Patients who had radiotherapy after resection cannot be analysed in this way as they must all have been survivors of surgery in order to proceed to radiotherapy and the results would therefore be distorted. One-month mortality in the no primary anti-tumour treatment group was 38.7% for 'other treatment', 47.4% for 'no treatment' and 43.7% for the whole group.

Table 6.2   One Month Mortality by Type of Treatment.

	Total number	Deaths at one month No.	%
Primary anti-tumour treatment			
Resection (± RT/CT)			
Resection only	1104	353	32.0
Resection + radiotherapy	29	Not applicable	
Resection + chemotherapy	8	1	12.5
Resection + radiotherapy + chemotherapy	2	Not applicable	
Radiotherapy/Chemotherapy (no resection)			
Radiotherapy alone	725	76	10.5
Chemotherapy alone	31	8	25.8
Radiotherapy + chemotherapy	12	2	16.7
No primary anti-tumour treatment			
Other treatments			
By-pass	60	30	50.0
Insertion of tube + exploratory surgery	479	163	34.0
Insertion of tube only	523	205	39.2
Exploratory surgery	120	61	50.8
Treatment to metastases	6	1	16.7
No treatment	1581	750	47.4
TOTAL	4680	1650	35.3

Table 6.3

When subdivided by sex, the 1-month mortality is seen to be consistently lower for females than for males in all treatment groups, except one in which the numbers were extremely small.

Table 6.3 One Month Mortality by Type of Treatment and Sex.

	Males			Females		
	Total number	Deaths at one month No.	%	Total number	Deaths at one month No.	%
Primary anti-tumour treatment						
Resection (± RT/CT)						
Resection only	548	185	33.8	556	168	30.2
Resection + radiotherapy	13	Not applicable		16	Not applicable	
Resection + chemotherapy	3	0	0.0	5	1	20.0
Resection + radiotherapy + chemotherapy	0	Not applicable		2	Not applicable	
Radiotherapy/Chemotherapy (no resection)						
Radiotherapy alone	434	50	11.5	291	26	8.9
Chemotherapy alone	19	5	26.3	12	3	25.0
Radiotherapy + chemotherapy	7	2	28.6	5	0	0.0
No primary anti-tumour treatment						
Other treatments						
By-pass	41	22	53.7	19	8	42.1
Insertion of tube + exploratory surgery	287	98	34.1	192	65	33.9
Insertion of tube only	310	132	42.6	213	73	34.3
Exploratory surgery	80	42	52.5	40	19	47.5
Treatment to metastases	3	0	0.0	3	1	33.3
No treatment	875	423	48.3	706	327	46.3
TOTAL	2620	959	36.6	2060	691	33.5

Table 6.4

As would be expected, these results simply reflect the judgement of the clinicians, as survival was much better in the curatively treated patients, both at 1 and 5 years. Nevertheless, occasional 5-year 'cures' were seen with both surgery and radiotherapy even when the treatment was intended to be palliative. It must be emphasised that these results do not provide a valid comparison between surgery and radiotherapy, as the histological and site composition of these groups differs greatly (see Tables 5.2 and 5.3).

Table 6.4 Age Adjusted Survival Rates (%) for Primary Anti-tumour Treatment: Curative v Palliative.

	Total number	One year	Five year
Resection (± RT/CT)			
[a] Curative	949	42.3	15.0
[b] Palliative	194	10.6	1.1
Radiotherapy/Chemotherapy (no resection)			
[c] Curative	353	28.2	6.5
[d] Palliative	415	7.8	0.3

Note : Letters in square brackets refer to lines on figure 6.4.

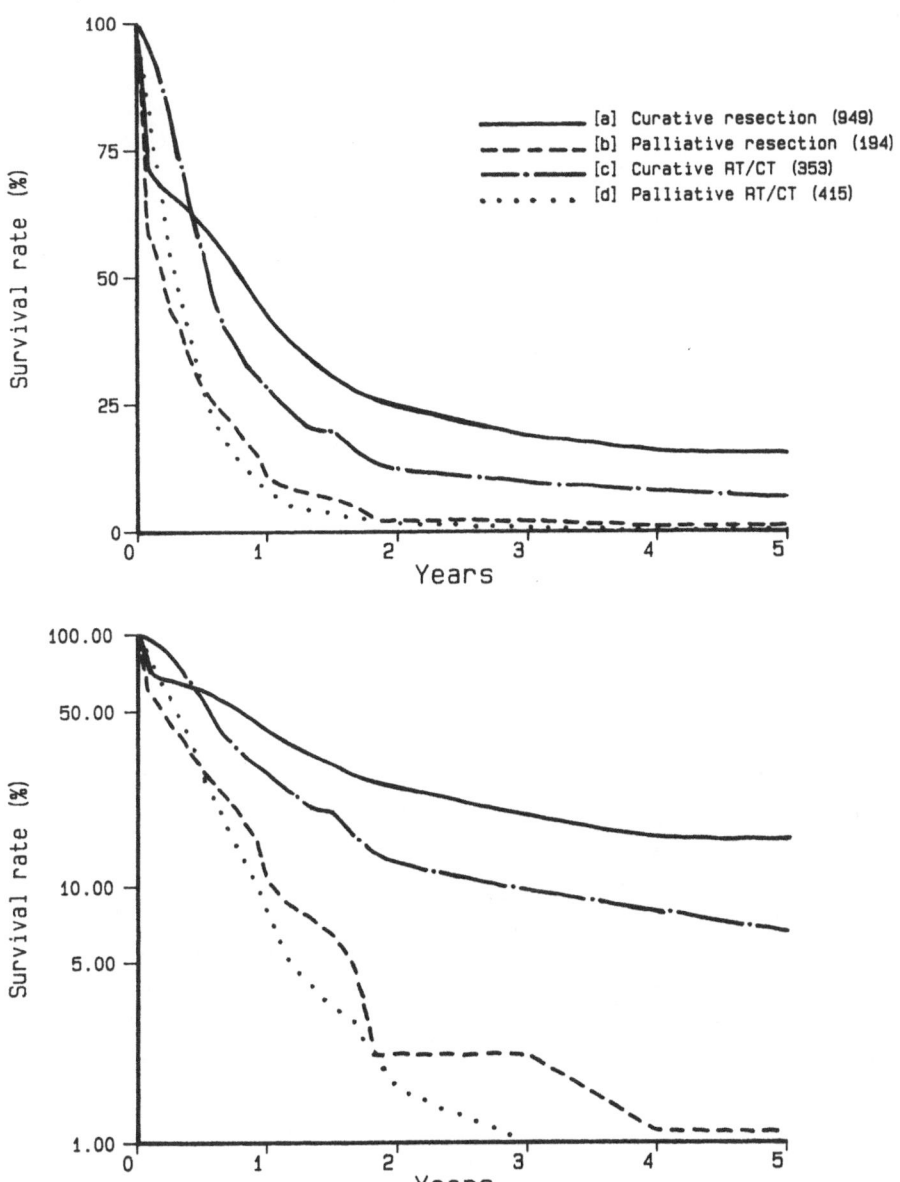

Figure 6.4 Primary Anti-tumour Treatment (PATT): Curative v. Palliative.

Table 6.5

These results again show a better survival rate for females in all the primary anti-tumour treatment groups, at both 1 and 5 years, with the exception of the 1-year results for palliative radiotherapy/ chemotherapy.

Table 6.5   Age Adusted One Year and Five Year Survival Rates (%) for Primary Anti-tumour Treatment: Curative v Palliative by Sex.

	Males			Females		
	Total number	One Year	Five Year	Total number	One Year	Five Year
Resection (± RT/CT)						
Curative	456	38.6	10.1 [a]	493	45.7	19.3 [b]
Palliative	108	9.6	0.0 [e]	86	11.9	2.5 [f]
Radiotherapy/Chemotherapy (no resection)						
Curative	214	23.5	4.1 [c]	139	35.3	10.1 [d]
Palliative	246	8.6	0.0 [g]	169	6.8	0.7 [h]

Note : Letters in square brackets refer to lines on Figure 6.5 (1-2).

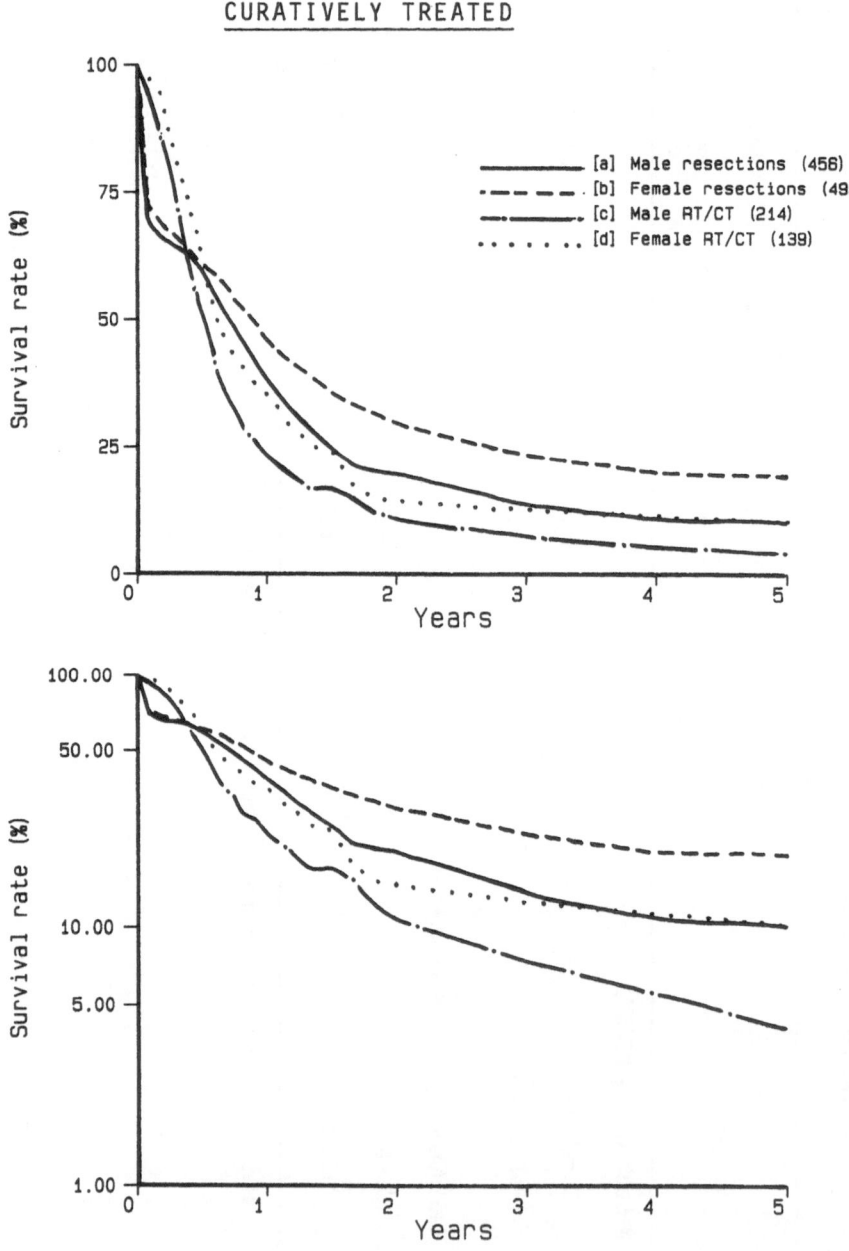

Figure 6.5.1 PATT: Curative by Sex.

PALLIATIVELY TREATED

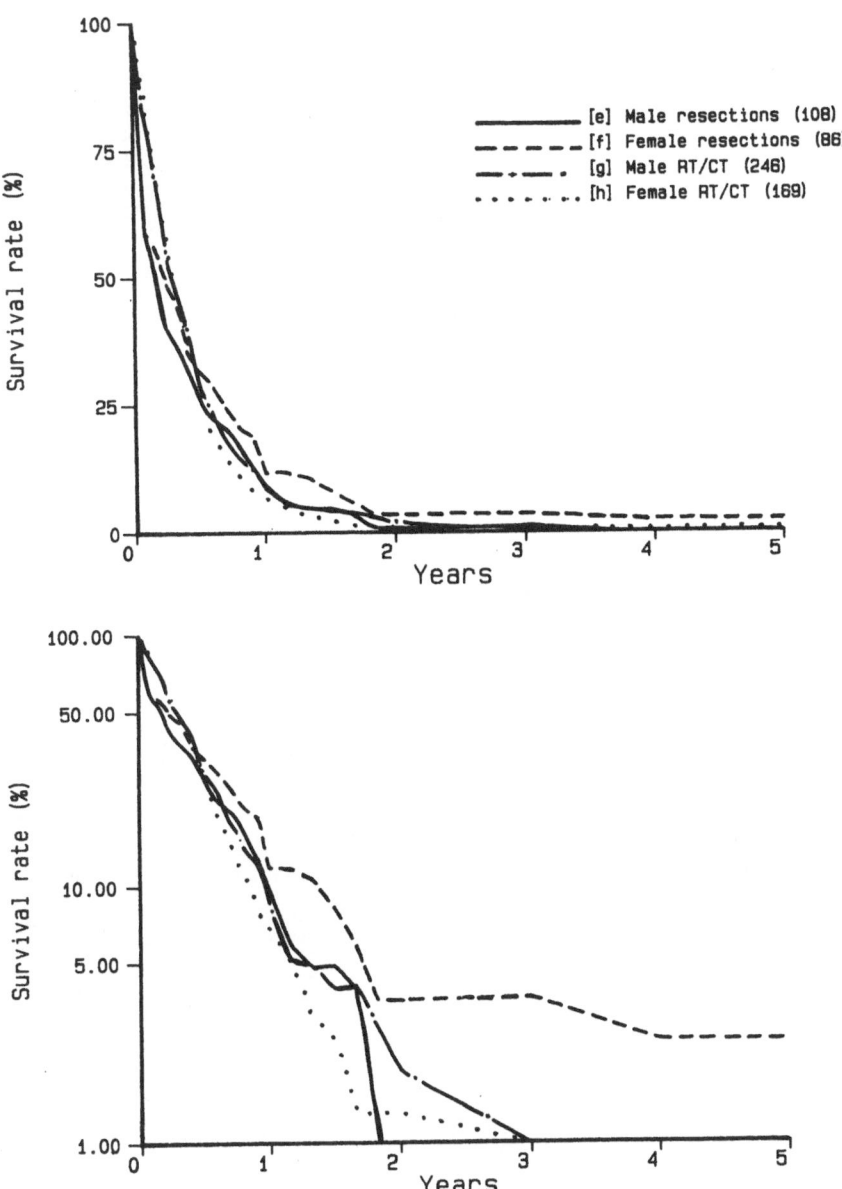

Figure 6.5.2   PATT: Palliative by Sex.

Table 6.6

Long-term survival is undoubtedly better with squamous tumours than with any other histology, but it is perhaps surprising that it was better with anaplastic tumours than with adenocarcinomas. In fact, 5-year survival was very rare in adenocarcinomas and was confined exclusively to patients having a curative resection. It is not possible to determine whether patients treated by curative resection were generally fitter or had earlier tumours than those treated by curative radiotherapy, so a direct comparison of these groups may not necessarily be valid.

Table 6.6   Age Adjusted One Year and Five Year Survival Rates (%) for Primary Anti-tumour Treatment: Curative v Palliative by Major Histological Groupings.

	Squamous cell ca.			Adenocarcinoma			Anaplastic		
	Total number	One year	Five year	Total number	One year	Five year	Total number	One year	Five year
Resection (± RT/CT)									
Curative	806	43.7	16.9 [a]	86	39.6	2.7 [b]	40	25.8	5.7 [c]
Palliative	149	11.0	1.5	20	15.4	0.0	20	5.1	0.0
Radiotherapy/Chemotherapy (no resection)									
Curative	284	29.5	6.4 [d]	6	0.0	0.0 [e]	24	21.6	5.0 [f]
Palliative	271	8.9	0.5	16	6.5	0.0	33	9.5	0.0

Note: Letters in square brackets refer to lines on Figure 6.6.

Resection (+ or - RT/CT)

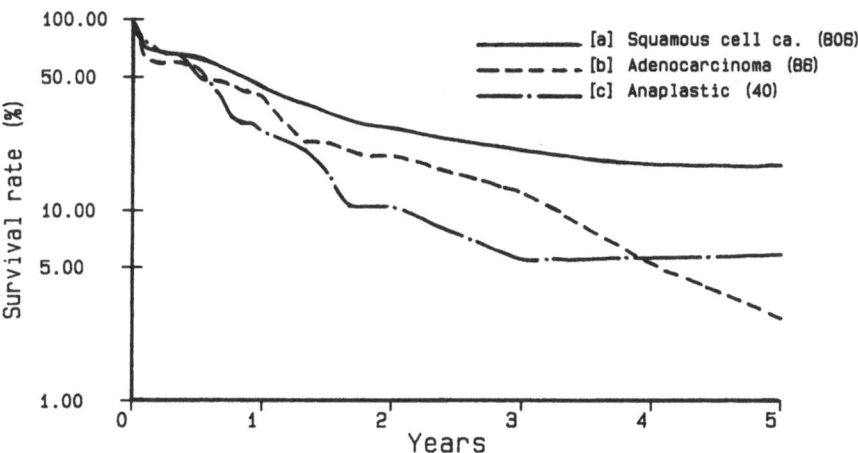

Radiotherapy and/or Chemotherapy (no resection)

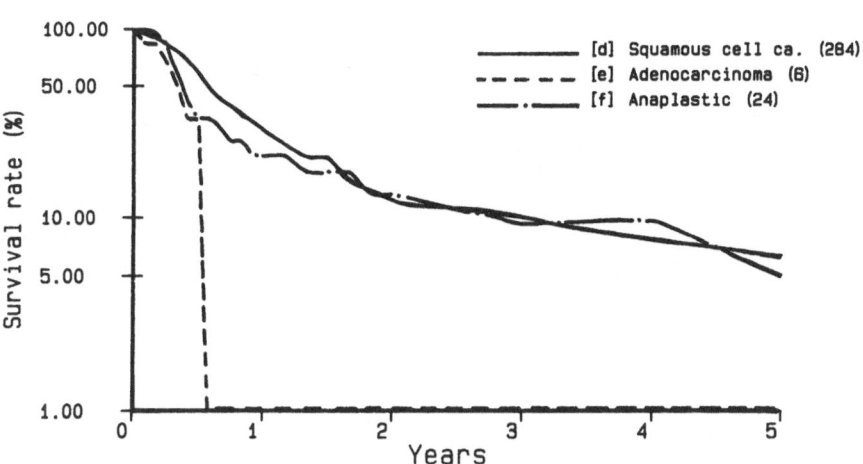

Figure 6.6   Curative Resection or Radiotherapy by Histology.

Table 6.7

Contrary to some statements in the literature, the prognosis following curative resection was as good for tumours in the middle third
as for those in the lower third.   The surgical complexities of remov-
ing the upper third of the oesophagus, however, mean that resection
was used less for tumours of this site, and the survival was less
than for radiotherapy, although again the groups may not be strictly
comparable.

Table 6.7 Age Adjusted One Year and Five Year Survival Rates (%) for Primary Anti-tumour Treatment: Curative v Palliative by Known Site.

	Upper third			Middle third			Lower third		
	Total number	One year	Five year	Total number	One year	Five year	Total number	One year	Five year
Resection (± RT/CT)									
Curative	38	21.5	8.6 [a]	355	45.4	15.3 [b]	520	42.3	15.8 [c]
Palliative	8	0.0	0.0	68	12.0	0.0	113	10.9	2.0
Radiotherapy/Chemotherapy (no resection)									
Curative	126	36.9	13.2 [d]	170	20.1	2.2	47 [e]	35.6	5.5 [f]
Palliative	82	6.4	0.0	221	9.5	0.6	89	5.9	0.0

Note : Letters in square brackets refer to lines on Figure 6.7.

Resection (+ or − RT/CT)

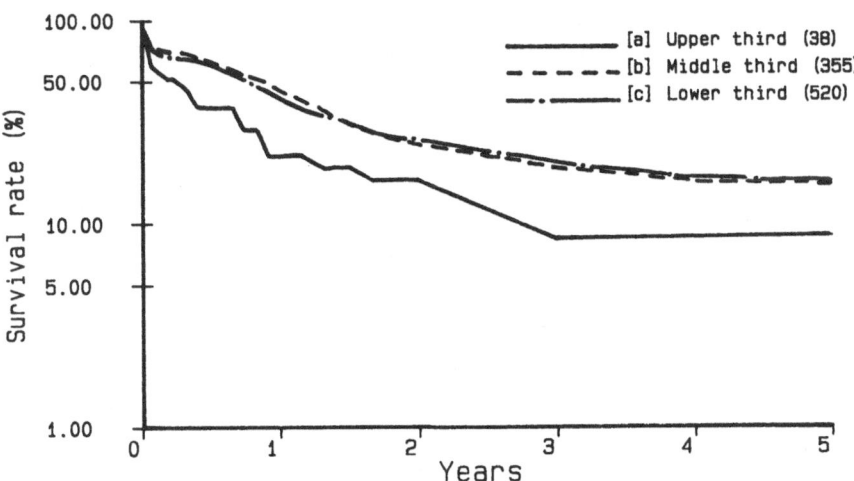

Radiotherapy and/or Chemotherapy (no resection)

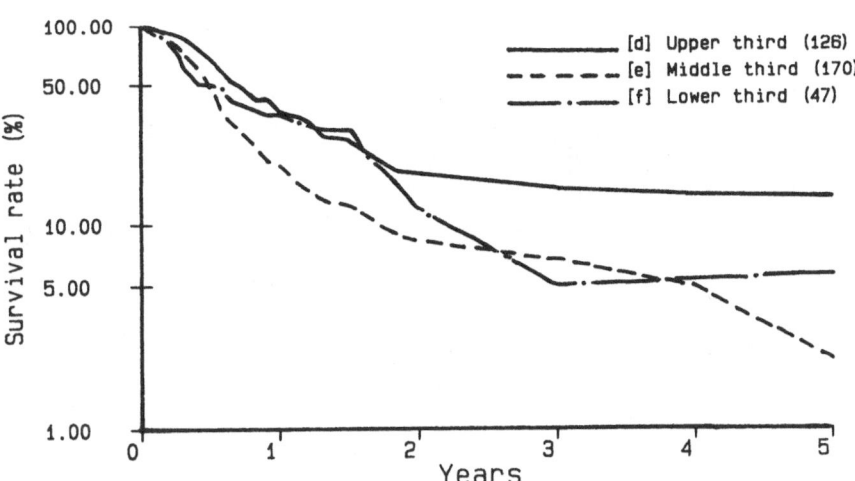

Figure 6.7   Curative Resection or Radiotherapy by Site.

Table 6.8

The better survival rate in females already noted is seen here to apply to all histological types having curative treatment. The non-resected adenocarcinomas and all anaplastic tumours have been excluded from the accompanying figures as the numbers are small.

Table 6.8 Age Adjusted One Year and Five Year Survival Rates (%) for Curatively Treated Patients: by Sex and Histology.

	Squamous cell ca.			Adenocarcinoma			Anaplastic		
	Total number	One year	Five year	Total number	One year	Five year	Total number	One year	Five year
Resection (± RT/CT)									
Males	353	39.0	12.4	62	41.8	0.0	29	28.5	4.1
Females	453	47.2	20.2	24	34.1	9.6	11	18.7	10.0
Radiotherapy/Chemotherapy (no resection)									
Males	161	24.0	4.7	5	0.0	0.0	18	23.1	0.0
Females	123	36.5	8.4	1	0.0	0.0	6	17.1	19.0

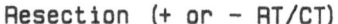

Resection (+ or − RT/CT)

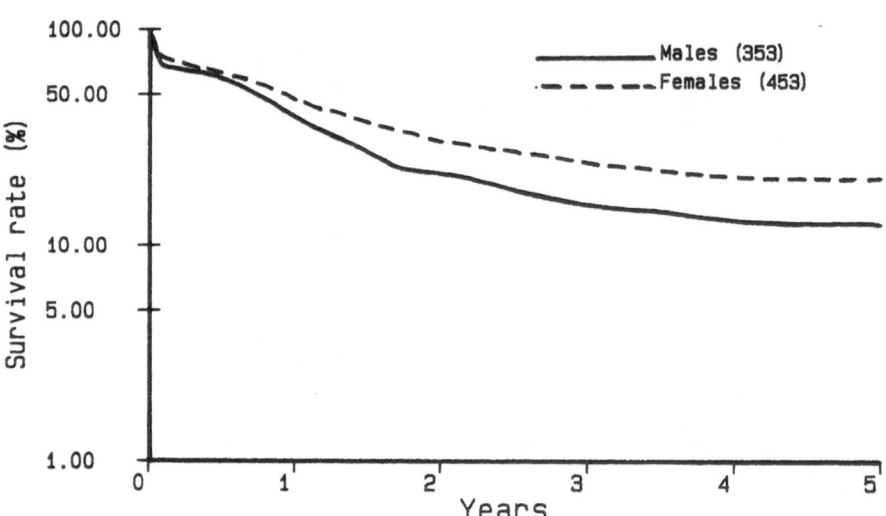

Radiotherapy and/or Chemotherapy (no resection)

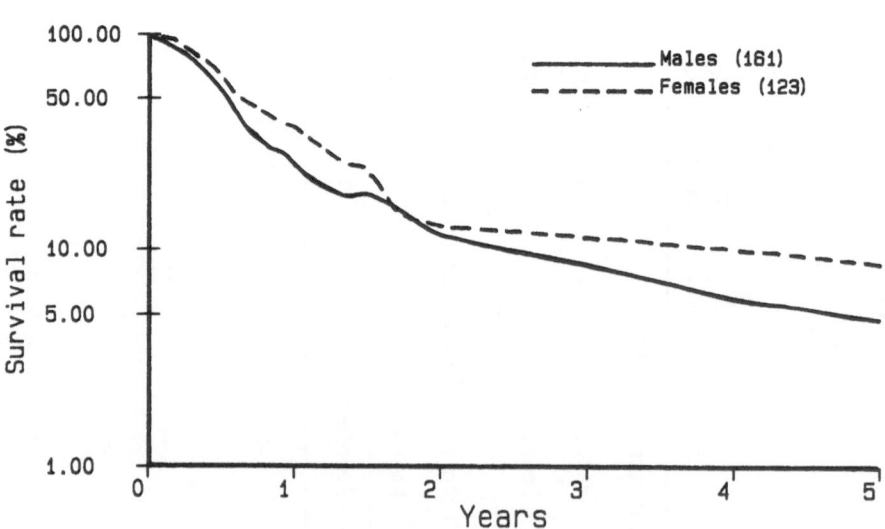

Figure 6.8.1   Squamous Cell Carcinoma.

Resection (+ or - RT/CT)

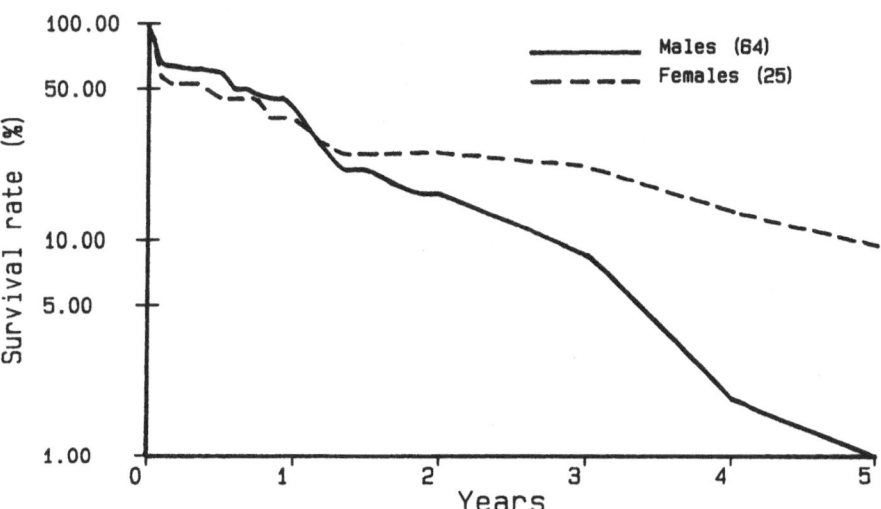

Figure 6.8.2   Adenocarcinoma: Resection (+ or - RT/CT).

Table 6.9

For curatively treated patients there is again a better survival for
females at all sites except one (middle-third tumours, not resected)
where the difference was not significant.

Table 6.9 Age Adjusted One and Five Year Survival Rates (%) for Curatively Treated Patients: by Sex and Known Site.

	Upper third			Middle third			Lower third		
	Total number	One year	Five year	Total number	One year	Five year	Total number	One year	Five year
Resection (± RT/CT)									
Males	16	12.9	0.0	156	38.5	9.2	266	40.9	11.5
Females	22	27.7	14.7	199	50.7	19.9	254	43.7	20.1
Radiotherapy/Chemotherapy (no resection)									
Males	66	25.4	7.2	108	20.3	2.4	34	27.8	4.2
Females	60	49.2	19.5	62	19.8	1.8	13	55.7	9.0

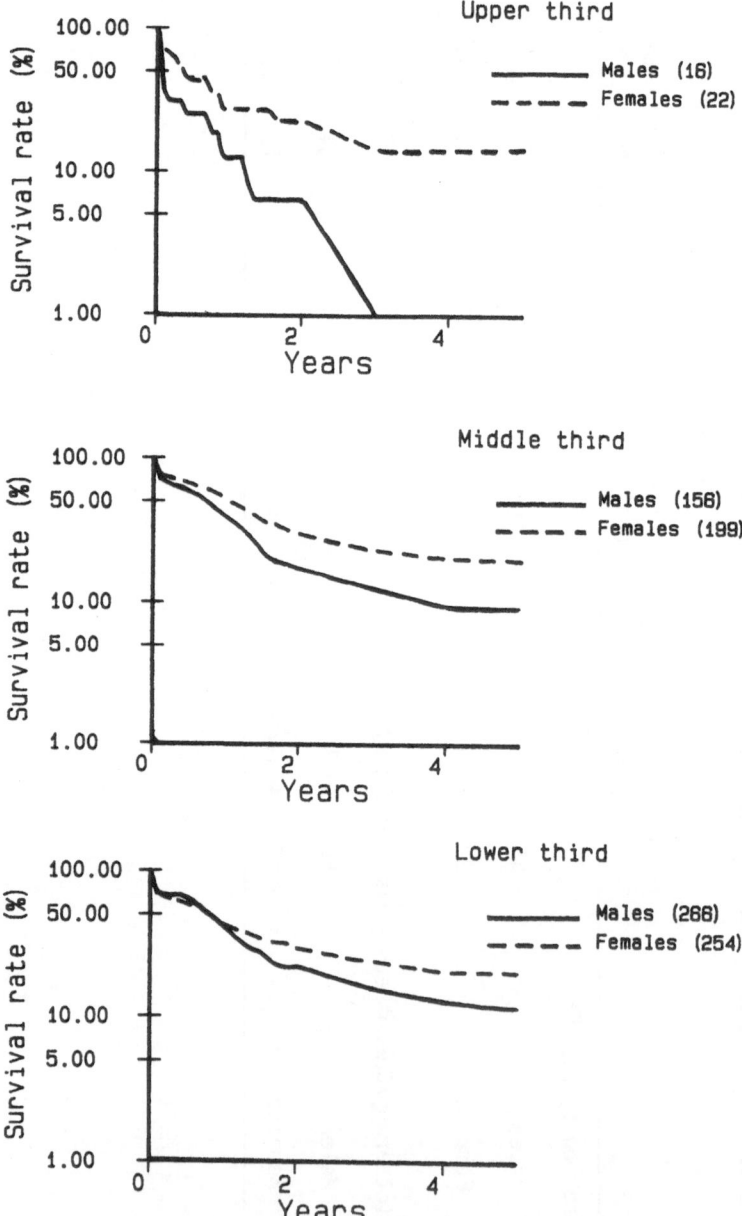

Figure 6.9.1 Curative Resection (+ or - RT/CT).

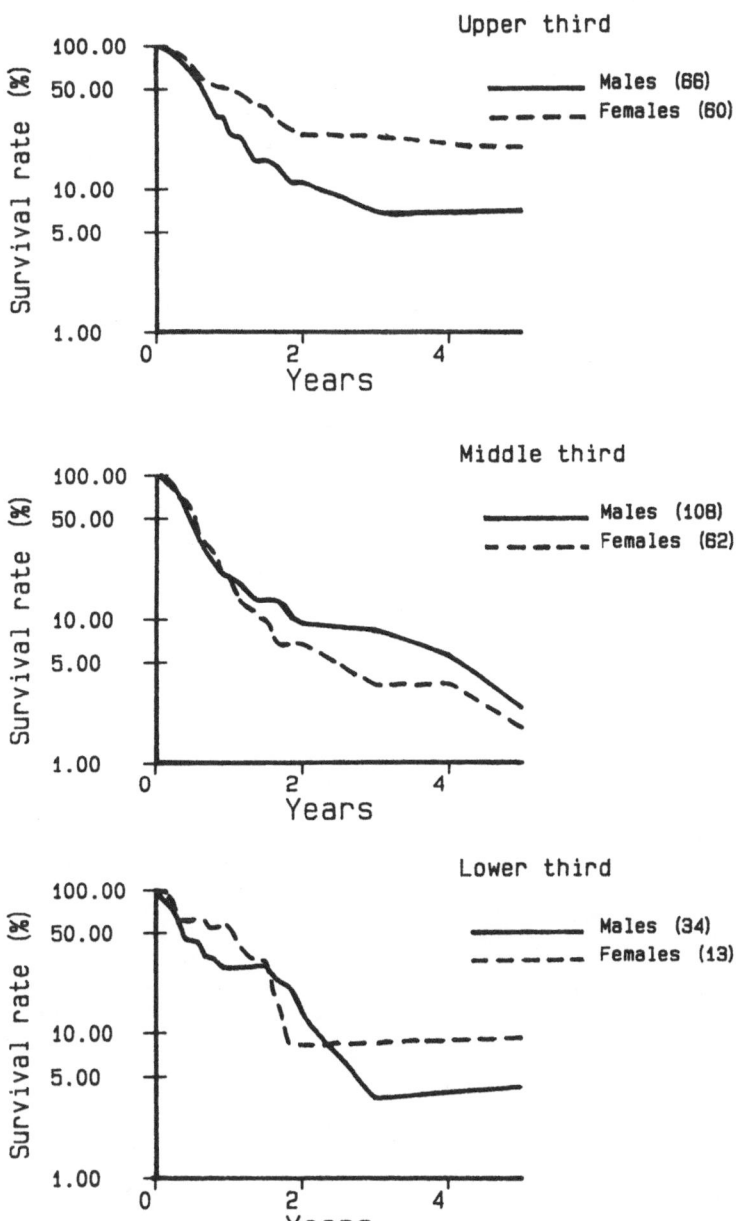

Figure 6.9.2   Curative Radiotherapy and/or Chemotherapy (no resection).

Table 6.10

Comparison of survival after curative treatment between the two decades shows no significant change in the results after resection, but shows a significant improvement in the results after radiotherapy for tumours of the upper third.

Table 6.10.1   One Year Survival Rates (%) for Curatively Treated Patients: by Site, Treatment and Decade.

	1957-66			1967-76		
	Total number	Crude rate	Age-adj. rate	Total number	Crude rate	Age-adj. rate
Upper third						
Resected cases (± RT/CT)	15	26.7	27.1	23	17.4	17.8
RT/CT (no resection)	70	27.1	28.0*	56	46.4	48.0*
Middle third						
Resected cases (± RT/CT)	149	41.6	42.6	206	46.1	47.4
RT/CT (no resection)	61	18.0	18.8	109	20.2	20.9
Lower third						
Resected cases (± RT/CT)	249	39.0	40.0	271	43.2	44.3
RT/CT (no resection)	14	28.6	29.9	33	36.4	38.1
Site unspecified						
Resected cases (± RT/CT)	20	30.0	31.0	16	37.5	38.7
RT/CT (no resection)	6	33.3	34.0	4	0.0	0.0
Total						
Resected cases (± RT/CT)	433	39.0	40.1	516	43.0	44.2
RT/CT (no resection)	151	23.8	24.7	202	29.7	30.8

Table 6.10.2 Five Year Survival Rates (%) for Curatively Treated Patients: by Site, Treatment and Decade.

	1957-66			1967-76		
	Total number	Crude rate	Age-adj. rate	Total number	Crude rate	Age-adj. rate
Upper third						
Resected cases (± RT/CT)	15	6.7	7.2	23	8.7	9.5
RT/CT (no resection)	70	5.7	6.8*	56	17.9	21.2*
Middle third						
Resected cases (± RT/CT)	149	14.1	15.7	206	13.1	15.0
RT/CT (no resection)	61	1.6	2.0	109	1.8	2.2
Lower third						
Resected cases (± RT/CT)	249	12.0	13.6	271	15.5	17.8
RT/CT (no resection)	14	0.0	0.0	33	6.1	7.8
Site unspecified						
Resected cases (± RT/CT)	20	10.0	11.6	16	0.0	0.0
RT/CT (no resection)	6	0.0	0.0	4	0.0	0.0
Total						
Resected cases (± RT/CT)	433	12.5	14.0	516	13.8	15.7
RT/CT (no resection)	151	3.3	4.0	202	6.9	8.4

Upper third: Radiotherapy/Chemotherapy

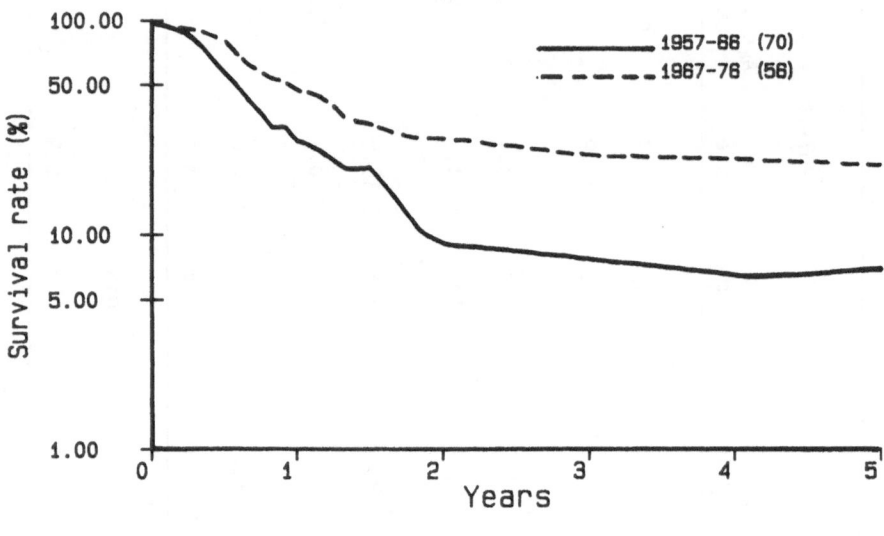

Figure 6.10.1

Middle third: Resection (+ or - RT/CT)

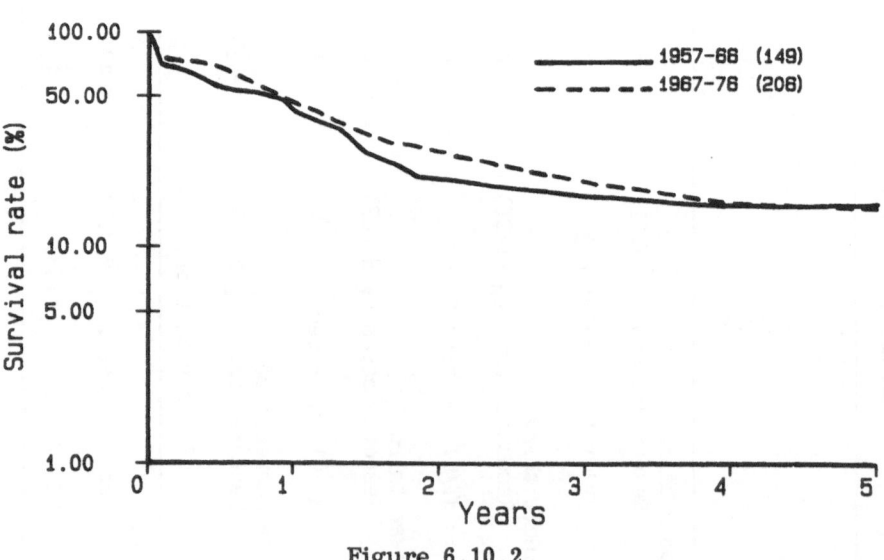

Figure 6.10.2

Middle third: Radiotherapy/Chemotherapy

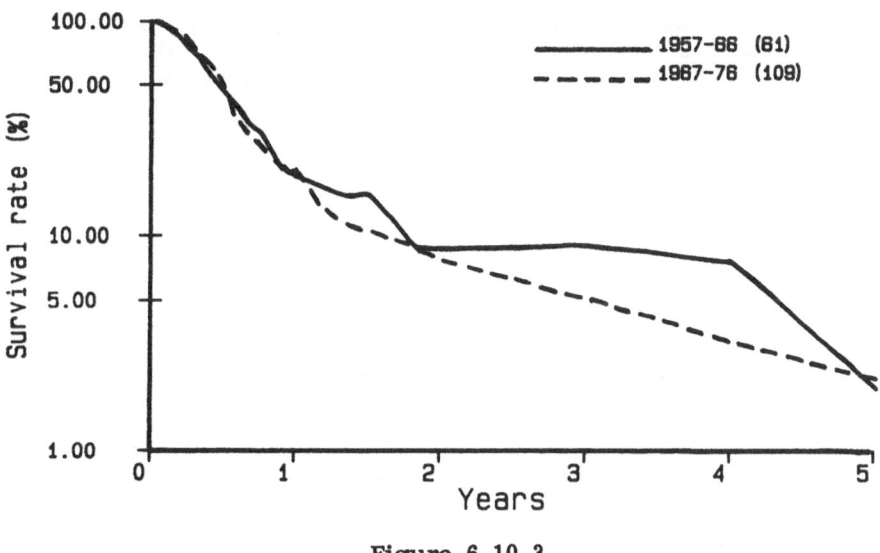

Figure 6.10.3

Lower third: Resection (+ or - RT/CT)

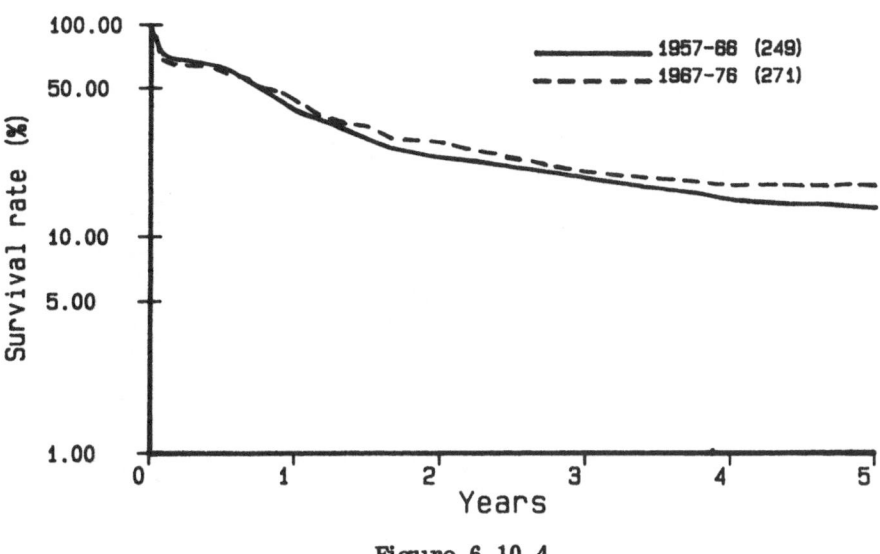

Figure 6.10.4

Table 6.11

Analysis of resected cases by histology and node status confirms what would be expected, namely that node-negative squamous tumours have the best prognosis. Nevertheless, some 5-year survivors are seen even with node-positive squamous tumours and even when the resection was thought to be palliative. Unfortunately a comparable analysis for patients treated by radiotherapy cannot be done, as their node status is not known.

Table 6.11 Squamous Cell Carcinoma. One Year and Five Year Survival Rates (%) for Resected Cases: by Node Status.

	Total number	One year rates		Five year rates	
		Crude	Age-adj.	Crude	Age-adj.
Curatively resected					
Node -ve	476	48.3	49.6	20.4	22.9
Node +ve	329	34.3	35.3	7.0	8.1
Node status not known	1	0.0	0.0	0.0	0.0
Palliatively resected					
Node -ve	48	10.4	10.7	2.1	2.2
Node +ve	101	10.9	11.2	1.0	1.1
Node status not known	0	-	-	-	-
Total					
Node -ve	524	44.8	46.0	18.7	21.0
Node +ve	430	28.8	29.6	5.6	6.4
Node status not known	1	0.0	0.0	0.0	0.0

<u>Table 6.12</u>

This table confirms that adenocarcinomas have a much worse prognosis than do squamous tumours, even when curative resection is performed, and no patient with involved nodes survived 5 years.

Table 6.12 Adenocarcinoma. One Year and Five Year Survival Rates (%) for Resected Cases: by Node Status.

	Total number	One year rates		Five year rates	
		Crude	Age-adj.	Crude	Age-adj.
Curatively resected					
Node -ve	48	43.7	45.2	4.2	4.9
Node +ve	38	31.6	32.5	0.0	0.0
Palliatively resected					
Node -ve	3	33.3	34.4	0.0	0.0
Node +ve	17	11.8	12.1	0.0	0.0
Total					
Node -ve	51	43.1	44.6	3.9	4.6
Node +ve	55	25.5	26.2	0.0	0.0

Table 6.13

As previously noted, anaplastic tumours have better results after resection than adenocarcinomas. Surprisingly, however, all the 5-year survivors had involved nodes - a finding which is as yet unexplained.

Table 6.13   Anaplastic Carcinoma. One Year and Five Year Survival Rates (%) for Resected Cases: by Node Status.

	Total number	One year rates Crude	One year rates Age-adj.	Five year rates Crude	Five year rates Age-adj.
Curatively resected					
Node -ve	21	19.0	19.6	0.0	0.0
Node +ve	19	31.6	32.5	10.5	12.0
Palliatively resected					
Node -ve	5	20.0	21.0	0.0	0.0
Node +ve	15	0.0	0.0	0.0	0.0
Total					
Node -ve	26	19.2	19.9	0.0	0.0
Node +ve	34	17.6	18.1	5.9	6.7

Table 6.14

This data shows generally that increasing age has a definite adverse effect on the long-term survival after surgery, but not after radiotherapy. It also confirms the better survival in females compared with males, as noted in previous analyses.

Table 6.14.1 Crude One Year and Five Year Survival Rates (%) by Age and Sex for Curative Resection.

Age group	Males			Females			Persons		
	Total number	One year	Five year	Total number	One year	Five year	Total number	One year	Five year
20 – 29	1	100.0	100.0	0	–	–	1	100.0	100.0
30 – 39	7	85.7	42.9	10	50.0	0.0	17	64.7	17.6
40 – 49	22	36.4	9.1	49	53.1	24.5	71	47.9	19.7
50 – 59	132	44.7	12.1	137	53.3	23.4	269	49.1	17.8
60 – 69	192	36.5	7.3	181	37.6	16.0	373	37.0	11.5
70 – 79	96	26.0	3.1	113	43.4	11.5	209	35.4	7.7
80 – 89	6	16.7	0.0	3	0.0	0.0	9	11.1	0.0
90+	0	–	–	0	–	–	0	–	–

Table 6.14.2 Crude One Year and Five Year Survival Rates (%) by Age and Sex for Curative Radiotherapy.

Age group	Males			Females			Persons		
	Total number	One year	Five year	Total number	One year	Five year	Total number	One year	Five year
20 – 29	1	0.0	0.0	0	–	–	1	0.0	0.0
30 – 39	7	42.9	14.3	6	83.3	16.7	13	61.5	15.4
40 – 49	14	28.6	14.3	20	20.0	0.0	34	23.5	5.9
50 – 59	56	21.4	1.8	32	31.2	6.2	88	25.0	3.4
60 – 69	166	11.4	1.2	81	19.8	4.9	247	14.2	2.4
70 – 79	51	21.6	2.0	38	34.2	10.5	89	27.0	5.6
80 – 89	15	26.7	0.0	4	75.0	25.0	19	36.8	5.3
90+	0	–	–	0	–	–	0	–	–

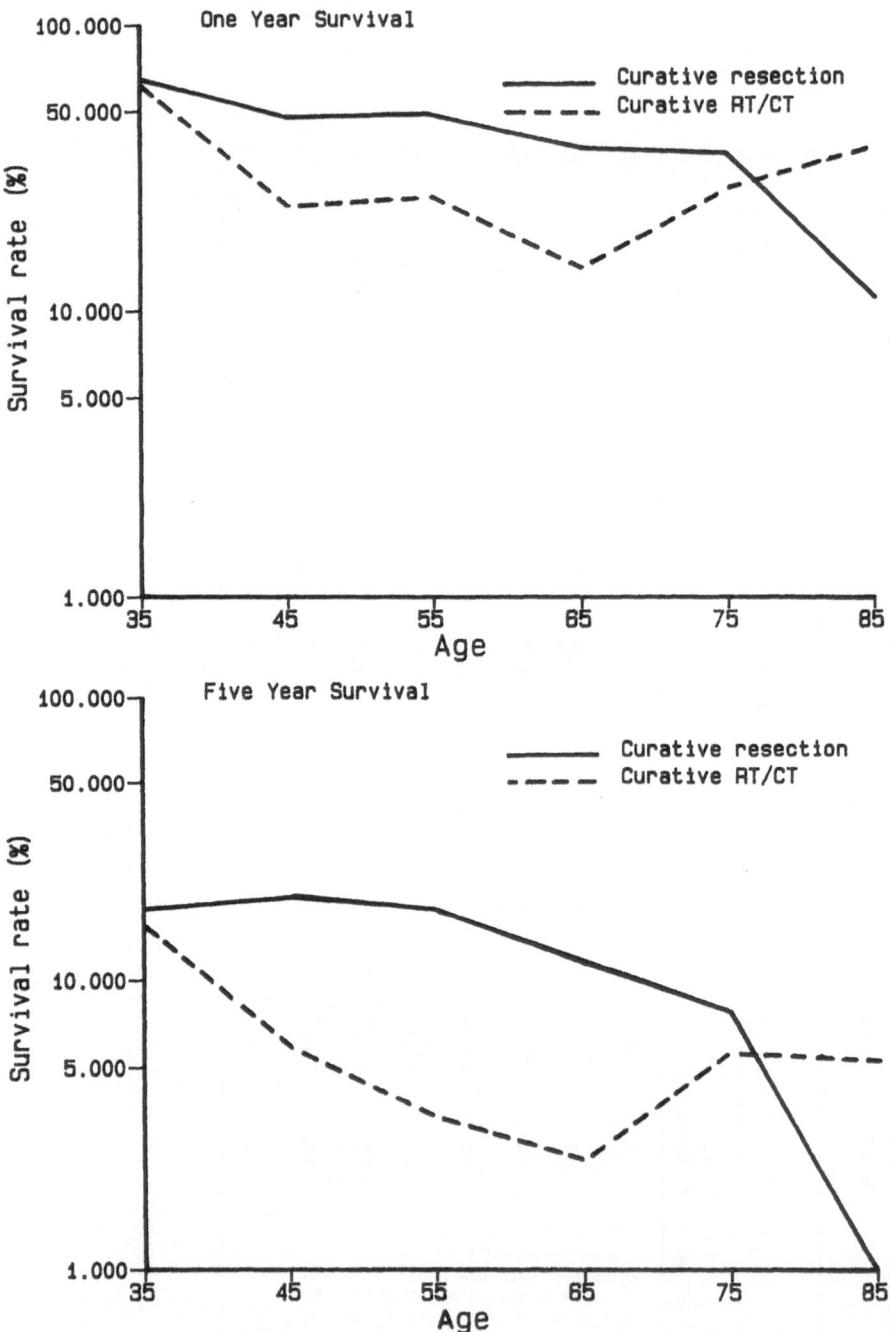

Figure 6.14   Curative Resection and Radiotherapy by Age.

Table 6.15

Of the 2769 patients who did not receive any primary anti-tumour treatment, less than 1% were alive at 2 years. This serves to emphasise that oesophageal carcinoma is a rapidly fatal disease but, paradoxically, may offer some hope in that it should be possible to test the efficacy of newer treatment regimes in a much shorter timescale than is required for most other forms of cancer.

Table 6.15 Age Adjusted Survival Rates (%): No Primary Anti-tumour Treatment.

	Total number	One month		One year		Two years	
		Number	Rate	Number	Rate	Number	Rate
[a] Other treatments	1188	728	61.4	37	3.3	5	0.5
By-pass	60	30	50.2	2	3.5	1	1.9
Insertion of tube + explor. surg.	479	316	66.2	10	2.2	0	0.0
Insertion of tube only	523	318	60.7	21	4.3	4	0.9
Exploratory surgery	120	59	49.3	3	2.6	0	0.0
Treatment to metastases	6	5	83.6	1	17.2	0	0.0
[b] No treatment	1581	831	52.8	60	4.1	16	1.2

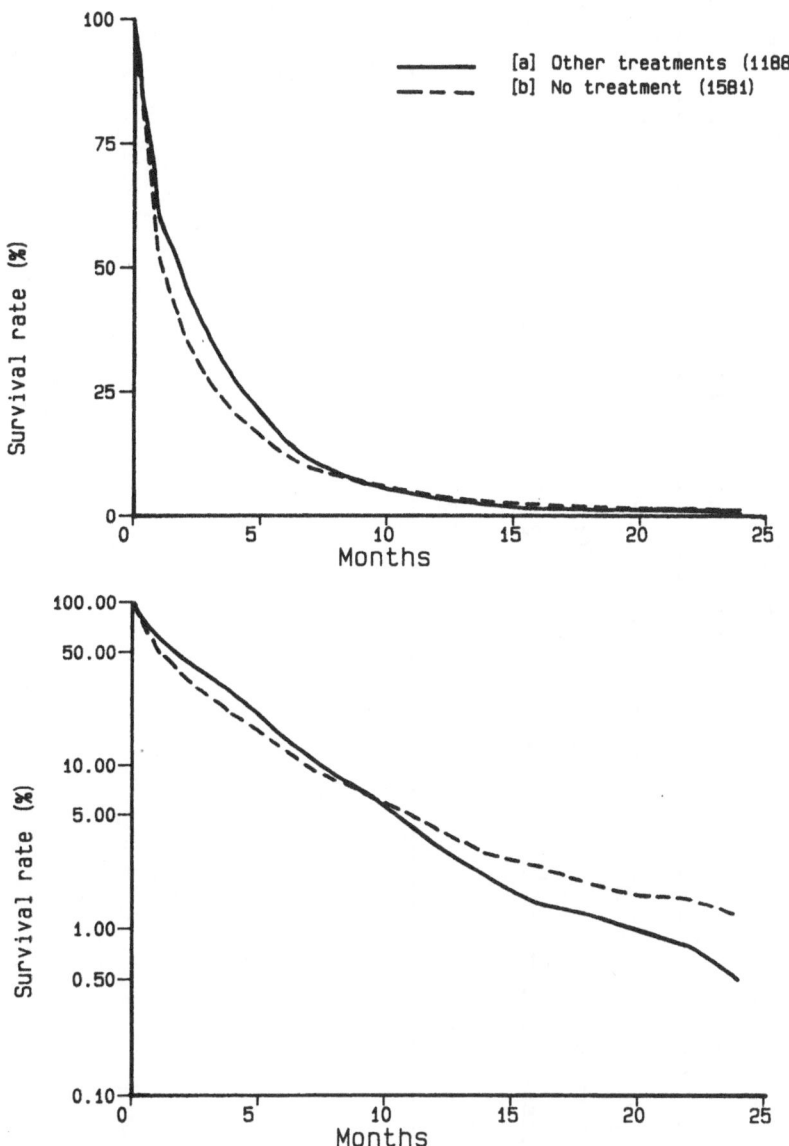

Figure 6.15   No Primary Anti-tumour Treatment.

Table 6.16

This gives the results by histology for patients who had 'other treatments' and shows that only one patient survived to 2 years.

Table 6.16 Age Adjusted Survival Rates (%): Other Treatment.

	Total number	One month		One year		Two years	
		Number	Rate	Number	Rate	Number	Rate
SCC	605	371	61.4	18	3.1	1	0.2
Adenocarcinoma	94	68	72.6	4	4.5	0	0.0
Anaplastic carcinoma	94	55	58.8	1	1.1	0	0.0
No histology	380	224	59.3	14	3.9	4	1.2

Table 6.17

This gives results by histology for patients having no initial treatment, although a few of these will have had treatment subsequently. Patients who had other histologies (e.g. adeno-squamous) are not included.

Table 6.17 Age Adjusted Survival Rates (%): No Treatment.

	Total number	One month		One year		Two years	
		Number	Rate	Number	Rate	Number	Rate
SCC	448	252	56.3	22	5.2	5	1.3
Adenocarcinoma	61	37	60.9	5	8.6	1	1.8
Anaplastic carcinoma	60	34	56.9	3	5.3	1	1.9
No histology	980	488	50.0	28	3.1	9	1.1

7

Atypical Tumours

In this chapter the clinical features of the 25 tumours known not to be carcinomas, and the three primary lymphomas, are tabulated, in order to allow the reader to make histology-specific analyses, if required.

We are indebted to Professor E.L. Jones for reviewing the slides of the three lymphoma cases.

Table 7.1 Clinical Table Showing All Cases of Lymphoma, Sarcoma and Other Rare Histologies.

Year of diagnosis	Age	Sex	Site	Histology	Presentation	Treatment	Fate
1959	67	M	M	Appearance suggestive of sarcoma	2 months dysphagia	None	D. 5 months Silico-tuberculosis, sarcoma oesophagus.
1961	61	M	L	Transitional cell ca.	2 months dysphagia & weight loss	Curative resection	D. 1 month Congestive cardiac failure
1962	75	F	L	Transitional cell ca.	Dysphagia	Exploratory surgery	D. 1 month Malignancy
1962	42	M	U	Low grade Liposarcoma	2 months dysphagia	Curative resection	D.15 yrs 11 mths Ischaemic heart disease
1963	78	M	Unsp.	Basal cell ca.		None	Found at P.M.
1963	66	F	U	Carcino-sarcoma	9 months dysphagia, weight loss, pallor, fatigue	None	D. 1 month Malignancy
1963	52	F	M	Fibro-sarcoma	2 months chest pain, dysphagia, anorexia, vomiting, weight loss, dyspnoea	Curative resection	D. 4 years 11 months Disseminated malignancy
1963	71	M	L	Myosarcoma	2 months dysphagia, anorexia, weight loss	Curative resection	D. 0 months Cerebral embolism, ischaemic heart disease
1966	53	M	Unsp.	High grade non-Hodgkin's lymphoma	18 months dysphagia	Curative resection	Alive & well at 20 years.

Table 7.1 (continued)

Year of diagnosis	Age	Sex	Site	Histology	Presentation	Treatment	Fate
1967	66	M	L	Carcino-sarcoma	Not known	Curative resection	D. 1 year 2 months Carcinomatosis
1968	65	M	M	High grade non-Hodgkin's lymphoma	6 months dysphagia, weight loss	Thoracotomy, Souttar's tube & curative radiotherapy	D. 11 years 0 months Myocardial infarction - no evidence of malignancy
1968	42	F	L	Non-Hodgkin's lymphoma	28 years dysphagia	Souttar's tube	D. 0 months Disseminated malignancy
1970	73	F	M	Pseudosarcoma	3 months dysphagia & local pain	Palliative resection	D. 4 months Malignancy
1970	71	F	L	Transitional cell ca. with basal cell	Dysphagia	Curative resection	D. 1 year 0 months Disseminated malignancy
1971	60	M	M	Leiomyosarcoma	2 months dysphagia	Souttar's tube	D. 2 months Malignancy
1971	60	F	M	Probably sarcoma	6 months vomiting	None	D. 0 months Malignancy
1972	78	M	Unsp.	Leiomyosarcoma	2 months dysphagia	Celestin tube	D. 2 months Malignancy
1972	63	M	M	Pseudosarcoma	2 months dysphagia, profound weight loss	Palliative resection	D. 1 month Carcinomatosis
1972	73	F	L	Carcino-sarcoma	Haematemesis	Mousseau-Barbin tube	D. 0 months Malignancy

Table 7.1 (continued)

Year of diagnosis	Age	Sex	Site	Histology	Presentation	Treatment	Fate
1973	82	F	L	Pseudosarcomatous Ca.	6 months anorexia & weight loss	Curative resection	Died 8 years 1 month Cerebrovascular Accident
1973	71	F	M	Carcino-sarcoma	3 months dysphagia	Curative radiotherapy	D. 7 months Malignancy
1973	63	M	M	Carcino-sarcoma	Local pain, dysphagia, anorexia, weight loss	Curative resection	Alive and well at 12 years
1973	47	M	M	Melanoma	2 months cough, dyspnoea & weight loss	None	D. 0 months Carcinomatosis
1975	40	F	L	Fibrosarcoma	2 months dysphagia	Palliative resection & chemotherapy	D. 9 months Malignancy
1976	62	F	M	Low grade fibrosarcoma	12 months dysphagia, haematemesis & melaena	Curative resection	D. 0 yrs 0 mths Acute coronary insufficiency, ischaemic heart disease
1981	77	F	U	Leiomyosarcoma	5 months dysphagia	Curative radiotherapy	Alive and well at 4 years
1981	67	F	M	Carcinoid	18 months dysphagia	Curative resection	D. 2 years 5 months. Carcinomatosis
1981	50	F	L	Leiomyosarcoma	2 months dysphagia	Curative resection	D. 4 years 11 months Primary squamous Ca. trachea

Appendix 1

Birmingham and West Midlands Regional Cancer Registry

Cancer registries are of two kinds: hospital-based and population-based. The first registers all cases of cancer seen at one hospital or at a small group of hospitals; the second aims to record every case of cancer occurring in a defined population.

A1.1 BEGINNINGS

The Birmingham Cancer Registry can be said to have begun in the form of a hospital-based registry, when a clerical officer was appointed towards the end of 1935 to complete the forms requested by the Radium Commission. This commission, set up in 1929, had been empowered to purchase and distribute radium, as the best-known and most useful source of radiotherapy, to the major hospitals of the country to aid in the treatment of cancer. It had requested some information concerning the patients treated by radium in order to provide some feedback on the efficacy of the programme. In an attempt to establish the value of radium in relation to other forms of treatment - chiefly surgery - details of patients not treated by radium were also requested. Radiotherapists, as the users of radium, readily complied, but unfortunately surgeons were less ready to do so, as they felt no similar sense of obligation.

The person appointed to undertake the work of data collection in the Birmingham General Hospital and the Queen's Hospital (now the Accident Hospital) was Miss Joan Levi, a woman of great drive and energy, motivated by an overriding sense of the importance of the work. Many will remember her and the force of her character: the pressure she would bring to bear on individual clinicians to maintain as complete a record as possible. The Registry owes much to her effort, both in the early days and subsequently, for the strength of the foundations she laid and for much of the super-structure put upon them.

World War II saw the destruction of most of the records of the Radium Commission when their offices were bombed in 1944. The

Registrar General then took over the responsibility of collecting the data from hospitals. Though Miss Levi's diligence led to the inclusion in the files of every case of cancer, treated or not, the registry was what would nowadays be called hospital-based. With the advent of the Health Service in 1948 and the regionalisation of cancer services, the collection of similar data on a regional scale became possible, the regions being the units of administration, each based on a population of several millions.

A Regional Cancer (Co-ordinating) Committee was set up in this Region, as in others. A small sub-committee of four of its members (the Professors of Medicine, Surgery and Pathology and the Reader in Medical Statistics - Dr Waterhouse) was formed which recommended setting up a cancer registry. It was one of the first to be set up in the UK. It centralised the collection of data about cancer patients for the Region and undertook the responsibility of making returns to the Registrar General for the Region as a whole, rather than individually by hospitals. Thus each hospital provided information directly to the Registry, and the Registry to the Registrar General. This is now the pattern throughout the UK.

The Director (Dr Waterhouse) decided that the records should be kept in the original form as submitted to the Registry (together with any subsequent pathology and follow-up reports, etc) and also in coded form on punch cards (and later on computer) to facilitate retrieval of data and analysis. A standard set of forms was devised for the collection of the data, requesting rather more than the basic minimum required by the Registrar General. In addition to the basic identification and social data about the patient and the names of the clinicians and hospitals involved, a full description of the tumour, both macroscopic and microscopic, and of the treatment given, is recorded. Follow-up reports are added, together with details of any extension of the growth (recurrences or metastases), the development of fresh primaries, and descriptions of the treatment given. At this time, the International Classification of Diseases chapter for neoplasms was inadequate, so that it became necessary to design a completely new system of hierarchical and contingent codes.

Naturally the Registry was not immediately fully effective or complete. There was no form of compulsion to provide data, nor active encouragement in the form of a fee (as for the notifiable diseases) so the system depended on voluntary agreement, though the mechanics of the system were provided by registration clerks (some specially appointed) in the various hospitals. The year 1960 is generally considered, in radiotherapy centres, to be the year when close to 95% coverage was achieved, resulting at that time in a total of just over 15 000 new cases. Twenty years later the total of the new registrations was about 22 000 a year, the increase being partly due to the ageing of the population (whereby more people are now living into the older ages where cancer is more common), and partly to the increased incidence of certain kinds of cancer (chiefly lung, bladder and prostate).

It is not only hospitals which are involved in providing data for the Cancer Registry. Routinely, all pathology laboratories also provide copies of pathology reports referring to cancer; coroners and their pathologists supply information on the extent of the disease at autopsy; general practitioners are most helpful in providing information on follow-up, including recurrence or further treatment; and the Registrar General sends, for deceased residents of the region, copies of all death certificates containing any mention of cancer.

A1.2 AIMS

What is the purpose of cancer registration - of collecting and storing a vast amount of information on patients with a single disease (or rather, group of diseases) which number now, in the Birmingham Cancer Registry, close to half a million cases? It began as a record of patients treated in a specific way in order to evaluate that mode of therapy. It is still patient-based (or, more properly, tumour-based, because a patient with two distinct primary cancers has two registrations) and it can be - and is - used for the evaluation of treatment regimens, though in rather more sophisticated ways than before. As a population-based registry, however, it acquires another mode of usefulness, in an epidemiological sense. When it is possible, as now, to discuss and analyse data referring to almost every patient (98%) with cancer in a region of 5.2 million people (the largest in the UK), to localise the tumour itself and its degree of spread, as well as the patient's residence, his treatment and his fate, then the detailed impact of the disease on a representative community can be very fully described and measured. Furthermore, changes and trends in the interaction between disease and community (which is the subject matter of epidemiology) can be detected and monitored. To some extent this can be done by the Registrar General for the country as a whole from the returns he receives from each regional registry, but his data are necessarily limited by the strength of the weakest link in the chain of registries; some are very poor, but none has the wide range of data that Birmingham has, and this accounts for its inclusion in a number of international studies, often as the sole representative of the UK. The passion of legislators to change the boundaries of administrative units and sub-units has affected many internal sub-division of the West Midland Region but (fortunately and uniquely in the UK) has left its outer boundaries unchanged. Thus it is possible to study and compare the changing patterns of cancer in a single sizeable area over a period of about a quarter of a century.

Internally, appropriate statistical indices can serve to characterise the pattern of cancer, by site, sex, age group, geographical sublocation, etc with obvious relevance to the provision of adequate services for diagnosis, treatment, follow-up, terminal care, etc. Such statistics, if kept in a uniform fashion over a period of time, will also furnish indications of changes in the impact of the disease, necessitating alterations in the services provided. It is also possible by extrapolation, based on plausible assumptions, to predict the requirements for the future. At the same time, the changes observed in the pattern of disease can be set against other characteristics (for example, occupational, environmental or geographical) in order to serve the purpose of monitoring the effects of known carcinogenic agents, and of detecting potentially new hazards.

In addition to the information they provide for cancer services, and for the observation of changes in the impact of the disease, the same or similar statistics can be used for clinical purposes, to evaluate the efficacy of treatment, to compile data on the natural history of the disease, or to assess the role of early diagnosis programmes, and in teaching (both undergraduate and postgraduate).

Appendix 2
Standardised Rates

A2.1 STANDARDISED INCIDENCE RATES

The very steep increase in risk with increasing age, which is characteristic of nearly all cancers, makes the number of cases likely to occur in a given 'population' (or defined group of people) very sensitive to their composition by age. In consequence, if the population includes a relatively large proportion of the elderly, more cancer cases are likely to be found than in a younger population.

The most convenient summary of the incidence of cancer in a population is expressed by the overall rate - that is, the total number of cancers divided by the total number of people in the population. Thus, if there are 800 cases in a population of 200 000, the rate would be quoted as 4 per 1000, or 400 per 100 000; either form could be used. This defines what is often called the 'crude' rate, in contrast to the age-specific rates which would be obtained by subdividing both the population and the cases of cancer into age groups (either 5-year, such as 35-39, etc or 10-year, such as 30-39, or more usually 35-44) and calculating an incidence rate for each age group. Subdividing also by sex, the numbers of cases in some of the age groups will be rather small, and will thus lead to rates which may not be very representative.

It would avoid the problems of dependency on the age structure of a population if we could always use the same one - a 'standard population' of known and constant composition. But each individual population encountered in practice has its own constitution by age. If, however, the age-specific rates are calculated from that given population, and then applied to the standard population (age group by age group), to obtain the number of cases that would be expected to occur in the standard population if it had experienced the rates (at each age group) of the given population, then the total of the expected cases can be used to provide the analogue of a crude rate in the standard population. This rate is then known as the 'standardised rate' for the given population. The nature of the standard population also needs to be specified. In contemporary usage, especially in the field of cancer rates, the most commonly quoted standard population is the World Standard Population, which is a constructed population, originally due to Professor Segi of Nagoya University in Japan; it is designed as an intermediate between the populations of developing countries, which are characterised by a large proportion in the younger age groups, and the European type having a population more evenly divided by age.

The method of standardisation of incidence rates described above is known as the 'direct method' (as opposed to the 'indirect method', which has not been used in this book).

Table 1 illustrates the method of calculation described above. It refers to a population of European type, and shows the reduction in the overall rate because the World Standard Population is of a younger structure.

A2.2 SURVIVAL RATES

The simplest form of the survival rate at 1 year is merely the ratio, expressed in the form of a percentage, of those patients alive a year after their treatment began to all those who were treated (i.e. the survivors and those who died before a year had elapsed). This is known as the 'crude survival rate', since no attempt is made to allow for any other factors, such as the age or sex of the patient.

The same procedure is adopted for the second year, whereby the survival rate is calculated as the ratio of those alive 2 years from the start of their treatment to those alive at the end of 1 year (and thus eligible to embark on a second year).

The 2-year overall survival rate, calculated by what is known as the 'actuarial method', is then the product of these two rates. If 2 years have elapsed for all the patients treated, then this product is the same as the crude 2-year survival rate calculated as the number alive 2 years from the start of treatment, divided by the total treated.

In symbolic form, if P_0 = the number of patients treated, P_1 = the number of these alive at their first anniversary and P_2 = the number alive at their second anniversary, then S_1, the 1-year survival rate, is P_1/P_0, and S_2, the survival rate for the second year, is P_2/P_1. The overall survival rate for 2 years $(SR)_2$, is then S_1 x S_2 = P_1/P_0 x P_2/P_1 = P_2/P_0, which is the same as the crude 2-year survival rate.

In a corresponding manner, the 5-year survival rate, computed actuarially, is obtained by multiplying together five rates, $S_1 S_2 S_3 S_4 S_5$, each one probably obtained from successively decreasing totals of patients, but thus utilising the data available to better effect. In this book, a full 5-year period of follow-up has been available for all patients.

Table 1

Age group x	Given population (males) Nos. in population P_x	Nos. of cases of cancer C_x	Incidence rate per 100,000 I_x	Nos. in World Standard Population W_x	Expected cases in Standard Population E_x
0–4	14,146	6	42.4	12,000	5.1
5–14	37,096	7	18.9	19,000	3.2
15–24	35,972	11	30.6	17,000	5.2
25–34	33,319	18	54.0	14,000	7.6
35–44	31,848	34	106.6	12,000	12.8
45–54	27,038	102	377.2	11,000	41.5
55–64	25,162	280	1112.8	8,000	89.0
65–74	17,407	345	1982.0	5,000	99.1
75–84	6,545	196	2994.6	1,500	44.9
85+	867	45	5190.3	500	25.9
Total	229,400	1044		100,000	

$$I_x = C_x / P_x \times 100,000$$
$$E_x = I_x \times W_x \div 100$$

Hence Crude rate $= \Sigma C_x / \Sigma P_x = 455.1$ per 100,000

Standardised rate $= \Sigma E_x / \Sigma W_x = 334.3$ per 100,000

Age Adjustment of Survival Rates

A group of elderly patients is unlikely to show as high a survival rate as another group, with the same condition and treated in the same way, whose average age is rather younger. Age is in fact one of the most important factors affecting survival rates. It can be allowed for in several ways, the most convenient of which is probably the Life Table Method.

The Life Table (Registrar General, 1979) gives, for each exact age x, and separately by sex, the number of individuals remaining alive (l_x) from a radix (initial number) of 100 000, all considered as having been born at the same time. The 'exact' age x is used, rather than the conventional usage (when a stated age refers to any day from the birthday itself to the day before the next birthday and is thus on average $x + \frac{1}{2}$), because the Life Table begins at birth which is exact age 0, and proceeds in yearly intervals from then.

Thus l_0 = 100 000, l_{65} = 70 426 and l_{70} = 56 715 (for males, from English Life Table No. 13, based on the 1971 Census). This means that out of 70 426 (= l_{65}) men alive at the exact age of 65, 56 715 (= l_{70}) are still alive 5 years later at the age of 70; for them, therefore, their 5-year survival rate would be l_{70}/l_{65} = 0.8053, or 80.53%.

Since ages are conventionally grouped into five consecutive years, a similar 5-year Life Table Survival rate for males in the age group 65-69 would be obtained from

$$\sum_{x=70}^{74} l_x \Big/ \sum_{x=65}^{69} l_x$$

which in fact works out to be 251361/326216 = 0.7705, or 77.05%.

The Life Table summarises the effect of all causes of death. For a group of, say, 100 patients in the age group 65-69, we would therefore expect 100 x 0.7705, which is 77.05 of them, to be alive 5 years later, if they were to experience the normal pattern of mortality. Taking the actual number who were in this age group at the time treatment began and had survived 5 years to be say, 30, then the crude 5-year survival rate for this group would be 30/100 = 30%, while the age-adjusted rate would be 30/77 = 38.94%, because only 77 would be expected to live for 5 years (from the Life Table).

This adjustment has been made for only a single age group. The same procedure can be extended very easily to cover the entire age range, and is most simply done by computing, from Life Table survival rates calculated as above, the total number of patients expected to be alive 5 years later, by adding together the separate expectations from each age group. The actual number of survivors, divided by this total of expected survivors, then gives the age-adjusted survival rate. Clearly, an exactly analogous procedure can be used for periods other than for 5 years, e.g. 10 years, 1 year, etc.

A more refined method uses the same principle but proceeds a year at a time, and uses the actuarial method for combining successive one-year age-adjusted survival rates over long periods. This means that the survival rate for the first year is calculated as the ratio of the number of patients who are alive on their first anniversary of the start of treatment, to the number of these same patients who would be expected to be alive after the lapse of 1 year, calculated by the use of the Life Table applied to the composition of the group of patients by age and sex. The number expected to survive for a second year is then calculated from the Life Table applied to the actual survivors, by sex and age (at the end of the first year). This number is then the denominator for obtaining the age-adjusted survival rate for the second year, using the number actually surviving to the end of the second year as the numerator. The method is repeated for each successive year, so that the adjustment for age is applied only to the actual survivors, and the 5-year age-adjusted survival rate is the product of the first five such rates. This is the method which has been used in this book.

A2.3 NUMERICAL ILLUSTRATIONS

Suppose that in the original example the number of patients initially treated (P_0) is 500, and that the number (P_1) surviving at their first anniversary is 250, then the 1-year crude survival rate (S_1) is P_1/P_0 which is 250/500 or 50%. If the number who are alive at their second anniversary is $P_2 = 150$, then the survival rate (S_2) for the second year is $P_2/P_1 = 150/250$ which is 60%. Thus the 2-year survival rate $(SR)_2$ is 150 out of the original 500, which is 30% and is the same as S_1 x S_2.

Excerpt from English Life Table No. 13 1970-72

x	l_x	x	l_x
65	70 426	70	56 715
66	67 994	71	53 570
67	65 400	72	50 335
68	62 648	73	47 038
69	59 748	74	43 703

For the age group 65-69, the expected (Life Table) 1-year survival rate is obtained by advancing the age group 1 year, to 66-70. The sum of the l_x figures for 66-70 gives the numerator of the fraction, and the sum for 65-69 gives the denominator. The computation is then the same in principle for each age group. For each successive year of survival, the actual survivors are reallocated to 5-year age groups and the same 1-year Life Table rates used for the calculation of expected numbers of survivors.

If 100 of the 500 patients in the example above were in the age group 65-69, and 55 of them survived to their first anniversary, the adjustment would be made as follows

$$\sum_{x=66}^{70} l_x \Big/ \sum_{x=65}^{69} l_x = \frac{312\ 505}{326\ 216} = 0.9580$$

0.9580 is the expected 1-year survival rate for this age group. Thus of 100 patients, 95.8 would be expected to be alive 1-year later. In fact, there were 55 survivors, for which the adjusted rate would be 55/95.8 = 57.4%, to be compared with 55/100 = 55%.

$$\sum_{x=67}^{71} l_x \Big/ \sum_{x=66}^{70} l_x = \frac{298\ 081}{312\ 505} = 0.9538$$

0.9538 is the expected 1-year survival rate for the next year, for a group now aged 66-70 to survive to be 67-71. The actual number of survivors was 55, of which 52.46 would be expected to survive (= 55 x 0.9538). If there were 42 survivors to their second anniversary, then their adjusted rate would be 42/52.46 = 80.06% for this second year, compared with 76.36 (42/55) unadjusted.

For the 2-year period, the number expected to survive out of 100 patients would be 100 x 0.9580 x 0.9538 = 91.37, and 42/91.37 = 45.97, to be compared with an unadjusted rate of 42/100 = 42%.

This example has been confined to a single age group. In practice, the expectations for each age group would be added together to give an overall expected number of survivors to 1 year, or 2 years, etc and the actual total of survivors at the same anniversaries would be set against these figures, to provide the appropriate age-adjusted survival rate. It is important that the calculation of expected survivors through each year is based on the actual age distribution of the survivors setting out on that year.

Appendix 3
Census and Inter-censal Populations

Census Populations

Age group	1961 Male	1961 Female	1971 Male	1971 Female	1981 Male	1981 Female
0 – 4	197,503	186,117	227,630	216,040	161,235	153,258
5 – 9	178,969	169,599	227,795	216,275	182,613	171,329
10 – 14	202,284	192,481	201,965	188,635	222,358	210,100
15 – 19	184,530	174,739	185,205	172,755	221,139	212,165
20 – 24	156,434	153,019	196,325	191,220	188,297	182,806
25 – 29	157,459	148,001	178,735	171,685	172,722	168,484
30 – 34	168,437	157,978	162,285	151,685	189,871	186,703
35 – 39	177,925	172,734	153,805	146,300	170,271	165,674
40 – 44	165,040	163,243	163,330	156,220	153,561	147,602
45 – 49	170,271	165,531	169,100	166,690	145,155	140,950
50 – 54	160,698	159,293	153,425	155,030	151,150	147,434
55 – 59	140,234	144,231	150,505	152,175	150,467	153,718
60 – 64	105,608	126,437	131,035	142,180	127,040	137,956
65 – 69	74,420	103,551	101,235	122,225	111,703	129,287
70 – 74	52,717	80,945	62,540	97,790	82,747	111,231
75 – 79	33,306	57,846	35,615	68,055	50,660	83,823
80 – 84	17,795	33,571	18,275	41,375	21,706	50,999
85 – 89	6,256	13,374	6,930	18,775	7,599	22,987
90 – 94	1,084	3,045	1,790	5,600	1,972	7,685
95 +	123	518	275	1,060	383	1,769
All ages	2,351,093	2,406,253	2,527,800	2,581,770	2,512,649	2,585,960

Inter-censal Populations

Age group	1966 Male	1966 Female	1976 Male	1976 Female
0 – 4	212,567	201,079	183,400	172,400
5 – 9	203,382	192,937	225,200	213,000
10 – 14	202,124	190,558	228,400	215,600
15 – 19	184,868	173,747	197,700	189,400
20 – 24	176,379	172,119	180,100	172,900
25 – 29	168,097	159,843	197,400	191,200
30 – 34	165,361	154,832	177,600	169,500
35 – 39	165,865	159,517	157,000	150,100
40 – 44	164,185	159,731	152,200	145,600
45 – 49	169,686	166,111	157,600	152,400
50 – 54	157,061	157,161	162,100	161,700
55 – 59	145,370	148,203	146,200	150,700
60 – 64	118,321	134,309	134,300	144,800
65 – 69	87,828	112,888	110,600	131,300
70 – 74	57,628	89,367	76,600	107,800
75 – 79	34,461	62,951	41,100	76,900
80 – 84	18,035	37,473	19,400	45,600
85 – 89	6,593	16,074	7,200	21,500
90 – 94	1,437	4,323	1,900	7,100
95 +	199	789	400	1,700
All ages	2,439,447	2,494,012	2,556,400	2,621,200

References

Bradford Hill, A., *Principles of Medical Statistics*, 8th edn, The Lancet, London (1966)

International Classification of Diseases, 9th revision, WHO, Geneva (1977)

Registrar General, *Census 1961, England and Wales*, County Reports, Table 6, HMSO, London (1963)

Registrar General, *Census 1971, England and Wales*, County Reports, Table 8, HMSO, London (1973)

Registrar General, *Life Tables: Decennial Supplement: 1970–72, England and Wales*, Series DS No. 2, HMSO, London (1979)

Registrar General, *Census 1981, England and Wales*, County Reports, Part 1, Table 6 (series CEN81 CR), HMSO, London (1982)

Registrar General, *Census 1981, England and Wales and Scotland. Persons of Pensionable Age, Great Britain*, Table 2, HMSO, London (1983)

Registrar General, *Census 1981: Key Statistics for Local Authorities: Great Britain*, HMSO, London (1984)

Waterhouse, J.A.H., *Cancer Handbook of Epidemiology and Prognosis*, Churchill Livingstone, London (1974)